# e-Clinical Governance

## A guide for primary care

Edited by

**Louise Simpson**

and

**Paul Robinson**

Radcliffe Medical Press

**Radcliffe Medical Press Ltd**
18 Marcham Road
Abingdon
Oxon OX14 1AA
United Kingdom

www.radcliffe-oxford.com
The Radcliffe Medical Press electronic catalogue and online ordering facility.
Direct sales to anywhere in the world.

British Library Cataloguing in Publication Data

A catalogue record for this book is available from the British Library.

ISBN 1 85775 595 2

Typeset by Joshua Associates Ltd, Oxford
Printed and bound by TJ International Ltd, Padstow, Cornwall

# Contents

# About e-clinical governance

*. . . the task is not so much to see what no one yet has seen, but to think what nobody yet has thought, about that which everyone sees . . .*

(Arthur Schopenhauer)

Clinical governance and health informatics – quality and computing. e-clinical governance is all about drawing together existing resources and expertise to help deliver exceptional patient care. This guide aims to show you how the information systems that are already present within most GP practices can help to enable and deliver clinical governance. Not only do we aim to show you that clinical governance and health informatics are partners in the same team, but how one can support the development of the other. In this guide, you will find more about teamwork, organisational learning and patient-focused care than about the (usually irrelevant) mess of wires within the grey box called the computer.

## Who is this book for?

You may be responsible for either information technology (IT) or clinical governance in your practice, primary care group or trust (PCG/T), or locality. You may be a GP, a nurse or another member of the team. You may be information proficient or you may prefer pen and paper to the mouse and screen. The common agenda is improving quality and improving patient care. This guide aims to give you a shared vision and a shared language to exploit the existing expertise and computing power to mutually support the informatics and the clinical governance agendas. Have fun!

## How to use this book

This book has been written as an easy-to-use, dip-in-and-out guide. It can be read from cover to cover, or you may choose to pick out one section and use that first. As well as being a guide to support the individual's knowledge development in both informatics and clinical governance in primary care, it can also be used as a teaching resource, either as background reading or you may use the 'bullet point' sections to prompt small group work.

# About the contributors

**Jane Cartridge** worked for several years in the health service followed by a stint at the Centre for Health Service Research at Newcastle University. Jane began working on PRODIGY during its early phases. During a three-year break, she worked as a freelance IT facilitator and creative writing tutor, and undertook an MA in creative writing. However, the SCHIN magnet got to work again and in 2001 she rejoined the PRODIGY team for Phase 3 evaluation.

**Dr David Graham** joined SCHIN as a clinical author in June 2001. He qualified from Nottingham University in 1987. He initially began his career in hospital medicine obtaining MRCP in 1991. David moved to general practice in Hexham and obtained MRCGP in 1993. He undertook a Diploma in Therapeutics in 1994 and has been the course leader since 2000. Whilst a GP, David was particularly interested and involved in teaching third and fifth year medical students and the training of GP registrars.

**Professor Ian Purves** is a former general practitioner and was appointed to lead the Sowerby Centre for Health Informatics at Newcastle (SCHIN) at its inception in January 1993. He is now Head of Centre and Professor of Health Informatics at Newcastle University. SCHIN is probably the largest centre of its kind in the world and is renowned for a broad agenda and for delivering quality beyond sponsors' expectations. Ian is interested in all aspects of health informatics, which he believes is strategically critical to the development of quality healthcare. His personal research interests are human factors within the consultation, decision support and the general philosophy of healthcare. Aside from his academic activities, Ian chairs, or is a member of, a number of national and international committees with respect to health informatics, in the belief that research should be put into practice.

**Dr Helen Raison** has worked at SCHIN since November 1996 and been closely involved with the development of PRODIGY. Helen moved her work base from Newcastle to Guildford at the end of 1999 and she is currently involved in all phases of PRODIGY. She previously held the role of Authoring Manager. Helen graduated from Newcastle Medical School. She has been active in curriculum development and teaching on the Health Informatics for Specialist Registrars course and the COGENT project.

**Dr Paul Robinson** has been a GP Principal for 17 years. He has 11 years' experience in medical education as a trainer and course organiser, and over the last five years has been involved in teacher training for medical educators. He has research interests in communication skills, knowledge use and knowledge structures. This has lead to his migration into the field of Medical Informatics. He is currently working on DoH funded research into the use of computers in the consulting room and is educational consultant to the NHS Appraisal Toolkit programme.

**Louise Simpson** joined the SCHIN team in October 1999 and leads the education and communications programme for PRODIGY (Release 1). She has 10 years' experience in primary healthcare, including a year's secondment to the NHS Executive, two years as a GP Computer Facilitator for Nottinghamshire FHSA and then as Group Manager for EMIS National User Group. Louise is an associate member of the Institute of Public Relations. She successfully achieved an MBA in 2000.

**Rob Wilson** has a degree in Sociology with an MSc in Social Research and is currently studying for his Doctorate. As well as being involved in the PRODIGY decision-support project from Phase 1, he has also been involved in the design and fieldwork of a number of research projects carried out at the Centre, including the RCGP's Scoping the EPR for Primary Care, the NHS Virtual Classroom project and leading the research on the Repeat Prescribing project. He is currently leading the work on the third phase of evaluation for PRODIGY (which includes user-centred design workshops, evaluation of system-generated interaction logfiles, questionnaires and clinical audit, interaction analysis of video data of doctors using the system in consultation, and the development of the training strategy) and Electronic Transmission to Pharmacy Pilot Evaluation research.

# Acknowledgements

We would like to thank all the team at the Sowerby Centre for Health Informatics at Newcastle (SCHIN), part of the University of Newcastle-upon-Tyne, especially the SCHIN training and communications team. Thanks also to Mike Sowerby and Dr Philip Leech from the Department of Health and to Steve O'Neill at the NHS Clinical Governance Support Team. It's been fun!

**Lou**
This book is dedicated to my lovely husband, Rob, and my terrific nephew and niece, Harry and Katie Simpson (aged 4 years and 3 months respectively).

**Paul**
To the patients who help me know how to be a doctor,
To the students who teach me how to be a teacher,
To Myra who shows me how to be myself.

# 1

# Introduction to e-clinical governance

*Louise Simpson*

---

**Key points covered in this chapter**

- Clinical governance and health informatics – partners in the same team

- The variety in health informatics

- What clinical governance leads say they want from informatics

- What can informatics offer clinical governance?

- The information age versus the industrial age of medicine

---

## So what's it all about?

The world has moved on since we first started talking about how to achieve this 'new' agenda of clinical governance. As primary care teams coordinate their activities in the delivery of effective practice, so informatics and the use of computer systems are important not only for 'doing' clinical governance but also for demonstrating that we are doing it. But clinical governance, like information management, is not just another thing to do, it is a way of working to do the thing we are in healthcare for – patient care.

e-clinical governance is about bridging the gap between computers and clinical governance, putting the patient at the heart of the process and about exploiting technology that is already available to most GPs in most practices. Informatics in clinical governance is much more than just a data collection function. Although quality data are important for the management and analysis of care quality, the electronic knowledge house on the clinician's desktop provides useful and useable access to evidence-based guidelines and clinical information, enabling medical practice to reflect medical science.[1] Electronic information systems do not and should not replace face-to-face ways of exchange; 'broadcast' is half the story, 'listen' and 'reflect' make up the other half.

Most clinical guidelines are produced on paper and if not locked away in the library, are only accessible via Internet searching, which is often inappropriate in the course of a typical general practice consultation. Most clinicians already have the power on their desktops to magic-up the required information – both reflective (in the form of the searches and audits) and proactive (in the form of clinical knowledge).

## What clinical governance wants from informatics

Research carried out by the University of Leicester[2] recently showed that 96% of PCGs and local health groups (LHGs) are developing a strategy for clinical governance. Clinical governance leads were asked to state and prioritise the support they needed to 'do' clinical governance and, after requesting more dedicated time, the next priority was to develop information systems. This suggests just how closely the delivery of information systems and technology has become linked with the delivery of the national agenda.

Further research carried out by the Sowerby Centre for Health Informatics at Newcastle (SCHIN) in 2001[3] showed similar results. If audit for audit's sake is a meaningless exercise, then computer use for its own sake is equally meaningless. It is only if there are clear benefits to the users that informatics becomes meaningful and clearly there *are* benefits to be seen in supporting the delivery of clinical governance.

## What can informatics offer clinical governance?

The uptake and use of computers in UK general practice has flourished – over 95% of practices now have a clinical computer system[4] and access to computer-based knowledge. In their 1995 research, Sullivan and Mitchell[5] reviewed the impact of computing on clinician performance in primary care. They found that all studies showed an improvement when the computer was used, citing access to 'scientific publications', decision support tools and computer-based prompts as a chief reason for this. Timpka et al.[6] reported that 67% of GPs in Sweden regarded their access to medical information as unsatisfactory, particularly in respect of therapy options. A key problem identified in their research was that GPs often worked 'far from essential sources of medical information'. Fox et al.[7] support this theme that most information has traditionally been locked away in paper-based libraries, usually far from the care intervention point: 'medical knowledge is traditionally disseminated via the publication of documents . . . Information technology offers to extend both modes of dissemination, via electronic publishing and virtual reality training'.

Walton et al.[8] also found that the quality of prescribing was significantly improved through clinicians' use of computer support tools. Furthermore, in a review of the effect of computer systems on prescribing errors published in *Bandolier*,[9] 60% of clinicians found benefit from clinical decision support systems in risk reduction. Evidence-based medicine provides a methodology for an individual practitioner to apply scientific knowledge to an individual clinical problem, bridging the gap between theory and practice.[10] Stonehouse and Pemberton[11] support this, stating: 'Location of the knowledge base is of crucial importance'.

## Why you don't need to worry about the stuff in the grey box of wires

If informatics is about using information to support and enable patient care, it is important to establish two principles. First, the 'technology', for most clinicians, is irrelevant. The old allegory is that you don't need to know how a car functions to drive safely from your base to your destination but you do need to know about putting the right fuel in and which pedals to press. It is the same with computers; programming languages are irrelevant for most of us, but using the right fuel (quality data) and navigating the pedals (the menus and functions of your software) will help you reach your destination a lot more smoothly.

The second principle is that computers are very good at doing routine jobs quickly and efficiently. For most people this means searching: for most practices, the days of pulling hundreds of sets of Lloyd George notes to run an audit are over. However, even the most paper-frugal practices think carefully about what their information requirements are likely to be and agree together what data will be captured on the practice system from patient encounters. Informatics is as much about teamwork and 'organisational learning' as any other element of general practice.

It is also worth thinking about the other benefits that the computer can bring to the practice, the clinician and the patient. 'Searches and audits' aren't the only type of information retrieval that clinical software can do quickly and efficiently. Later chapters will explore many aspects and applications in more detail, and you should find most – if not all – within existing GP computer software.

Patient expectations have changed too. An increasing number of households have a personal computer and patients are increasingly used to 'surfing the Net' for clinical information, some of it of dubious quality.

## The new information age

The industrial age has made way for the information age (*see* Figure 1.1), and consequently the implications for patients are emerging. Healthcare professionals no longer stand at the gateway to health information and knowledge, but the emphasis is on self-care and responsibility, supported by a partnership with the clinical team, rather than managed by a paternalistic relationship.

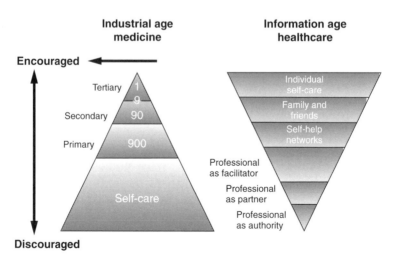

**Figure 1.1**  Changing patterns of healthcare. Adapted from Ferguson.[12]

Clinical governance can be seen as part of this paradigm shift and information and informatics can be a route to:

- enabling access to up-to-date clinical knowledge and evidence
- enabling effective use of extelligence (that domain of knowledge that lies outside the clinician's own head)
- facilitating reflection on activity and practice (mirrors)
- allowing us to demonstrate our excellence too (shop windows).

All are key aspects in the clinical governance programme.

The 'task' model of consultation (Figure 1.2) describes the tasks and roles of the patient, the clinician and the clinical computer system within the consultation. This 'triadic relationship' and its impact on clinical governance is covered in Chapter 3, but a look at the model reinforces the overlap between clinical governance and informatics – the language, meaning and focus are common to both. Ian Purves describes this as:

- exploring the story to categorise the problem, and understand the illness experience and patient health beliefs
- balancing the evidence of experience and up-to-date research findings using clinical information systems
- explaining professionally informed health beliefs to the patient
- enabling the patient to make an informed management decision cognisant of the benefits and risks of potential therapy, through possible shared computer interaction

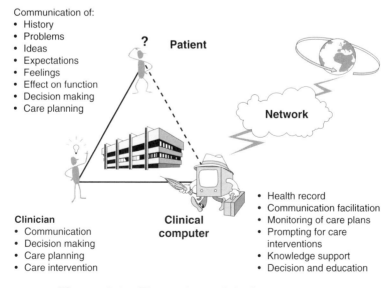

**Figure 1.2** The task model of consultation.

- engendering self-care through assessment of motivation and barriers, having realistic goals plus reinforcement of professional health beliefs over time
- incorporating prevention and health promotion through computer prompting
- enhancing the healing relationship between the individual and clinician
- making adequate electronic notes about the story to enable teamwork.

Later chapters look at concepts in clinical governance and health informatics, drawing a picture of how the domains overlap and how one supports, enables and facilitates the other. For proficient health informaticians, we hope to bring you some insight into the clinical governance agenda and for those with an interest in clinical governance, we hope to show how health informatics can help deliver the challenges in hand. But most of all, this book draws a picture of teamwork, organisational learning and how to manage the dynamic between disciplines to the mutual benefit of both, with easy-to-understand examples and practical guidance.

The shift from industrial to information age is acknowledged, as is the shift from patient to 'citizen'. Chapter 7 looks at the emerging e-health agenda from the patient's perspective and its role in clinical governance.

So can IT support clinical governance? Perhaps the question should be, can clinical governance be delivered without it?

# References

1  Donaldson LJ (2000) Clinical governance: a mission to improve. *Br J Clin Governance* **5**: 6–8.
2  University of Leicester (2000) Survey of the development of clinical governance in England and Wales. University of Leicester, Leicester.
3  SCHIN (2001) PRODIGY Phase III Survey. SCHIN, Newcastle.
4  University of Newcastle (2000) PRODIGY dissemination GP questionnaire. University of Newcastle, Newcastle.
5  Sullivan F and Mitchell E (1995) Has general practitioner computing made a difference to patient care? A systematic review of published reports. *Br Med J* **311**: 848–52.
6  Timpka T, Ekstrom M and Bjurulf P (1989) Information needs and information seeking behaviour in primary health care. *Scandinavian Journal of Primary Health Care* **105**(9): 105–9.
7  Fox J, Johns N and Rahmanzadeh A (1998) Disseminating medical knowledge. *Artificial Intelligence in Medicine* **14**: 157–81.
8  Walton RT, Gierl C, Yudkin P, Mistry H, Vessey MP and Fox J (1997) Evaluation of computer support for prescribing. *Br Med J* **315**: 791–5.

9   Bandolier (1999) Computer systems prevent errors. *Bandolier* **5**(6).
10  Robinson P (1999) Scarborough Vocational Training Scheme. www.scarbvts. demon.co.uk (accessed 4 May 2000).
11  Stonehouse G and Pemberton J (1999) Learning and knowledge management in the intelligent organisation. *Journal of Participation and Empowerment* **7**(5): 131–44.
12  Ferguson T (1995) *The Ferguson Report*. www.fergusonreport.com (accessed August 2001).

# 2

# Concepts in health informatics

*Ian Purves*

---

**Key points covered in this chapter**

- The history and background of computerisation in general practice

- The extent of computer use

- How is health informatics different to computerisation?

- Clinical data and information

- That's the theory, what about the practice?

---

## General practice computerisation

Health informatics is often considered to be the use of computers in the healthcare system. As you will see later in this chapter, it is much much broader than this, but many people do access health informatics through computerisation.

People come to health informatics through a variety of routes: for example, the total quality management activities of the late 1980s. However, the story of computerisation in UK general practice started much earlier, with a few keen GPs writing software programs to help them keep their registration data, run their repeat prescribing systems and send letters out to call patients for preventative services. These individuals were supported through a 'community of practice', the Primary Health Care Specialist Group of the British Computer Society and some through funding from the Micros for GPs scheme.

Computerisation remained light through the early 1980s until two suppliers – AAH Meditel and VAMP – offered their systems for free in exchange for the practices' pseudoanonymised data. These schemes eventually folded but they spawned a wider uptake of computers. From the new GP Contract in 1990, government funding became available for the purchase and maintenance costs of computers and an increasing number of practices acquired them. By 1996 most practices had a computer (*see* Figure 2.1).

## To what extent are the computers used in general practice?

We are all well aware, however, that there is a variability in how computers are used in primary care. Table 2.1 shows the progress in the use of computers from 1993 (note: 1993 data are practice based but 1996 and 2000 are individual GPs' responses).

So what does Table 2.1 tell us? It tells us that of the 96% of GPs who are computerised, 86% use them for clinical records. Furthermore 35% keep mainly electronic records (10% are paperless) and 33% use them in all consultations. It also shows that there is a general progression in utilisation

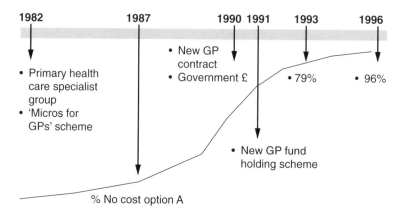

**Figure 2.1** Uptake of computers in UK general practice.

**Table 2.1** What GPs use their systems for in the UK

| Task | | Percentage of practices to use computer for task in 1993 | Percentage of GPs to use computer for task in 1996 | Percentage of GPs to use computer for task in 2000 |
|---|---|---|---|---|
| Clinical records | Partial | 42 ⎫ | 49.8 ⎫ | 51.5 ⎫ |
| | Partial, but eventually full | 19 ⎪ | 19.4 ⎪ | * ⎪ |
| | Full, retaining manual records | 29 ⎬ 90 | 15.8 ⎬ 91.5 | 24.3 ⎬ 85.1 |
| | Full, replacing manual records | – ⎭ | 6.5 ⎭ | 10.3 ⎭ |
| Repeat prescribing | | 94 | 91.3 | 99.8 |
| Audit | | – | 68 | 94 |
| Entry of clinical data during consultation | Some consultations | 32 ⎫ | 48 ⎫ | ** ⎫ |
| | All consultations | 44 ⎬ 66 | 33.1 ⎬ 81.1 | ** ⎬ 73.4 |
| Viewing clinical data during consultation | | 63 | 76.7 | 47.4 |
| Acute prescribing during consultation | | 58 | 72.9 | 90.6 |
| Use of computerised guidelines/ protocols during consultation | | 29 | 27.7 | 37 |
| Email | | – | 12 | 30 |

\* Respondents were asked specifically about the level of computerised records, and questions did not equate exactly to previous surveys.
\*\* The question did not differentiate between some and all consultations.

over the years. It is worth asking what are the major factors that hold GPs back from paperless practice?

Waring[1] (2000) identified these barriers as cost (71%) and legitimisation (47%). In autumn 2000, however, the GP Terms of Service Paragraph 36 was altered to legitimise paperless practice, so things may have changed. In addition, following 'legitimisation', the British Medical Association (BMA) and Royal College of General Practitioners (RCGP) produced advice on 'Good Practice Guidelines for General Practice Electronic Patient Records'.[2] What are the consequences? It appears there is a more

## Table 2.2

| Health informatics theme | What is it? |
| --- | --- |
| Generic computer skills | Interface skills: keyboard, mouse, pen and voice; common package skills; navigating the Web |
| Data management | Understanding collection and variability of health data; data quality assurance; transformation of clinical data with storage and communication |
| Organisational issues of information | Power and cultural issues resulting from the availability of information; understanding and practising within the wider NHS information environment; management information systems; the management of change and business process re-engineering; selecting/procuring clinical information systems |
| Confidentiality, security, legal and ethical issues of clinical data | Ethical framework; confidentiality; UK law and patient-based computer systems; risk assessment, security policies and security architectures |
| Communication | Authoring and reading of health records; coding: natural language, clinical nomenclature and classification; group working |
| Transforming clinical data into information and knowledge | Presentation and use of clinical information in patient management; using information in audit and clinical governance; research and development; epidemiology; medical statistics; using information to manage resources; knowledge management |
| Clinical decision making | Cognitive/narrative theory of clinical decision making; evidence-based medicine; guidelines; computer-assisted clinical decision support; shared decision making; image analysis, biological signal processing and pattern recognition |
| Continual learning with computers | Self learning – patient focused, 'just in time', distance and coordination; sources and retrieval of clinical information/knowledge |
| The patient–clinician–computer encounter | Clinical method; using a computer in the encounter; computer-assisted clinical methods |
| Clinical information systems | What is a clinical information system; architectural/technical/'workstation' considerations |
| Principles of health information system design | Communicating your requirements; iterative design methodologies; evaluation of health information systems; human computer interaction; standards; computer science technologies |
| Clinical knowledge engineering | Critical appraisal of publications; group dynamics for consensus; cognitive modelling of clinicians; methods of authoring knowledge bases |

rapid uptake of paperless or paper-frugal practice, which has also been influenced by PCG/Ts prioritising funding for computerisation.

# How is health informatics different to computerisation?

That is the background to general practice computerisation, but how is health informatics different? It is a *scientific* approach to information, which includes how we think, how data become information and knowledge, how we communicate in clinical practice, how we represent data, information and knowledge in computers, how we learn, how computers can support clinical practice and so on (*see* Table 2.2).

# Clinical data and information

It is important in a book on e-clinical governance that we understand the basic health informatics issues of observing and measuring clinical data, the issues of recording and communicating these data and then how they might be presented to someone.

## *Observation and measurement*

Clinical data have a surprising variability and inaccuracy embedded within clinical observations, measurement and techniques.[3] These potential problems originate from a number of sources:

- the patient's decision to seek care – his perception of himself as 'sick'; his definition of being 'sick enough'; socioeconomic barriers to care
- patient–clinician dialogue
- variability in the medical history – the patient's description of his illness; the clinician's selection of questions to ask (motivational bias, cognitive limitations, situational factors); patient psychological barriers to accurate information (fear of illness, guilt, falsification)
- variability of the physical examination[3,4]
- variability in interpreting investigation results – numerical data; image/pattern recognition; evidence of observer variability
- variability in defining the disease – advances in medical knowledge; variation in pattern recognition; tolerance of uncertainty by the clinician.

## Recording and communication

Communicating the content of a clinician–patient encounter is fraught with issues.[5] Fundamentally, the message, conversation or record has no meaning embedded in it – the receiver interprets this. Some of the issues that influence the meaning interpreted by the recipient are as follows.

- **Clinical vocabulary**, which can be used to convey precise medical concepts, but can simultaneously dehumanise the patient's story.[6] In addition, the words can be 'coded' either in human codes (i.e. English, French) or computer codes (e.g. Read, ICD10), and translation between these different coding systems can cause loss of the content – and meaning – of the message. Computer coding is one of the frustrating aspects of using clinical information systems. Codes are necessary because computers are too stupid to understand natural language and so we have to give them limited coding schemes. Some of these coding schemes are for classification (e.g. ICD10) and some just enable the nearest representation to natural language words, so-called nomenclatures (e.g. Read, SNOMED CT). Classifications are used to 'chunk' medical data for epidemiological reasons, and nomenclatures are to record patient data for clinical care. Using the wrong coding scheme can have a major impact on the medical record.
- Clearly the **grammar** that we use is relevant. From a computer perspective this means the headings we use under which we place codes and the codes/words (e.g. not, 'family history of') can modify the meaning of a word (e.g. diabetes) in close proximity. These computer semantics are among the hardest problem for the health informatician and the most frustrating for users when the computer is too stupid to understand the obvious.
- Another issue is the advantages/problems of **sharing** records between differing clinical disciplines – the perspective of each discipline is different and if not understood can cause confusion. For example, doctors describe things from their own perspective, whereas a nurse usually describes things from her own and often the patient's perspective too.

## Presentation of clinical information

The way that clinical data are presented can significantly impact on what meaning is placed on communication, which in turn can have significant impact on both clinical care and clinical governance. Is it a raw chunk of text? Is it generated through a computer query? Does it remain 'intact' with the rest of the words that make up the record of a clinical encounter?

# The role and challenge of electronic health records

The objective of the healthcare record is to support the aim of individual and population-based healthcare.* Fundamentally, it is based on the individual and is a contemporaneous list of observations about the individual's physical, psychological and social wellbeing.[7] The record is made by a selection of clinicians and should contain their thought processes, the context in which their observations were made and personal margin notes to assist with their delivery of care. The core purpose is communication.

Interestingly, despite the healthcare record having a clear focus to its purpose, there is a wide variability of the content and structure of healthcare records, on both an intra- and inter-professional basis. Perhaps the lack of availability of information from paper-based records has downgraded the role of the healthcare record to that of an '. . . *after the act . . . damn nuisance, no time for . . . personal memory jogging . . . medico-legal justification of management decisions . . .'*.[8]

With the advent of computerised healthcare records the problem of availability and legibility of paper records has been resolved. In fact, some have been worried that this accessibility and the old paper record paradigm will create a degree of misinformation.[9] However, accessibility within a new record paradigm will ensure that the healthcare profession can address the challenges to improve both the process and outcome of care.[10]

Only about 10% of clinical communication is via the health record, with most (around 50%) being verbal. This adds to the challenge of improving communication to improve clinical practice because failures in communication are the largest causes of error. It also raises the issue of the quality of the record, which is the substrate of audit and many forms of quality improvement. So aside from technological and clinical governance issues there is a large personal attitudinal education and cultural agenda.

The time has come to ensure that the content and structure of the healthcare record help clinicians achieve the mission of healthcare outlined. It is likely that, in primary care, doctors will need to change aspects of their clinical method.[11] The new healthcare record will introduce

* The aim of healthcare is to identify problems (whether they are presented or are asymptomatic) and to understand the impact of the illness on the individual, then resolve or ameliorate the problem to the patient's satisfaction, within the bounds of medical capabilities and society's resource limitations, while helping the individual cope with and manage his or her illness.

and maintain this method, and at the same time ensure that other professional groups will begin to work as an effective team with the patient.

## Clinical purposes

Practices currently require a patient record system that can be used to:

- assist in the clinical care of individual patients by:
  - assisting the author to structure his or her thoughts and make appropriate decisions
  - acting as an aide memoire for the author during subsequent consultations
  - making information available to others with access to the same record system who are involved in the care of the same patient
  - providing information for inclusion in other documents (e.g. laboratory requests, referrals and medical reports)
  - storing information received from other parties or organisations (e.g. laboratory results and letters from specialists)
- assist in the clinical care of the practice population by:
  - assessing the health needs of the practice population
  - identifying target groups and enabling call and recall programmes
  - monitoring the progress of health promotion initiatives
  - providing patients with an opportunity to contribute to their records.

## Non-clinical purposes

Practices also need a patient record system that can be used to meet administrative, legal and contractual obligations by:

- providing medico-legal evidence (e.g. to defend against claims of negligence or breach of service)
- providing legal evidence in respect of claims by a patient against a third party (e.g. for injuries, occupational diseases and in respect of product liability)
- meeting the requirements of specific legislation on subject access to personal data and medical records
- providing evidence of workload within a practice or a PCG
- providing evidence of workload to health authorities (e.g. to support claims and bids for resources)
- enabling the commissioning of community and secondary healthcare services
- monitoring the use of external resource usage (e.g. prescribing, laboratory requests and referrals).

### *Additional purposes*

Some practices also currently require a patient record system that can be used to:

- interact with a decision support/expert system
- support medical audit
- support teaching and continuing medical education
- enable:
  - epidemiological monitoring
  - surveillance of possible adverse effects of drugs
  - clinical research.

## So what needs to happen?

Fundamentally, for successful clinical governance activity there needs to be an improvement in patient record keeping. This is both a personal and organisational issue and involves changes in many areas – simply focusing on coding standards is not appropriate. Intelligent e-clinical governance informs clinicians about making best use of computer nomenclatures and using the best classification system to analyse the subsequent recording to generate meaningful clinical governance information.

## Other aspects of clinical information systems

Currently clinical information systems are focused on the Electronic Patient Record and the things you can do with it.

- Present patient data from the record intelligently on a screen to support the process of clinical practice.
- Present knowledge from external sources focused specifically on the needs of the clinician and patient within the consultation.
- Act as a focus for the clinician and the patient to aid debate on the next best actions.
- Act as a resource for personal and organisational learning by giving information for reflection and by presenting relevant knowledge during learning time.

# Knowledge management

As it stands, our information systems facilitate explicit knowledge* management. We might ask how this will progress. Will we be able to introduce a full knowledge management programme? As we have seen earlier, the record forms only 10% of clinical communication, and we know that the hard part of knowledge management is the management of tacit knowledge.** The nearest we get to the transfer of tacit knowledge is the use of narrative in a very specific context and the recipient interpreting the meaning. Those who are evangelical about evidence-based medicine might say this is not valuable. The rest of us know otherwise! So how do we facilitate the exchange of explicit knowledge (with clarity of its known effect using evidence-based techniques) and in the same context enable tacit knowledge interchange?

We need to understand the conversion processes between each form of knowledge.[12] These can be described as:

- tacit-to-tacit (*socialisation*) – where individuals acquire new knowledge directly from others
- tacit-to-explicit (*externalisation*) – the articulation of knowledge into tangible form through dialogue and story telling
- explicit-to-explicit (*combination*) – combining different forms of explicit knowledge, such as that in documents or on databases
- explicit-to-tacit (*internalisation*) – such as learning by doing, where individuals internalise knowledge from documents into their own body of experience.

## *Flood of information, drought of knowledge?*

The primary challenge of explicit knowledge is managing its volume to ensure its relevance. A common problem facing organisations is information overload, as the levels of explicit knowledge become so overwhelming that they cannot be appropriately filtered. Most organisations are currently focused on the management of explicit knowledge (heightened by the vast Inter/intranet resource of transient knowledge). But as organisations make advances in knowledge management, they realise that managing tacit knowledge is even more strategic, albeit more

---

\* 'Can be expressed in words and numbers and can be easily communicated and shared in the form of hard data, scientific formulae, codified procedures or universal principles.'[12]

\*\* 'Is highly personal and hard to formalise. Subjective insights, intuitions and hunches fall into this category of knowledge.'[12]

difficult. For tacit knowledge, the challenge is to formulate the knowledge into a communicable form in the first place.

The knowledge management domain needs to cover the above four processes, but in addition it has three other functional requirements.

- *Intermediation* – the process of brokering knowledge transfer between an appropriate knowledge provider and knowledge seeker.
- *Cognition* – the function of systems to make decisions based on available knowledge.
- *Measurement* – referring to all knowledge management activities that measure, map and quantify corporate knowledge and the performance of knowledge management solutions. This function acts to support the other functions, rather than to actually manage the knowledge itself.

Fundamentally, clinical information systems need to progress towards systems that are intermediate between the clinicians' and patients' knowledge needs and support the transfer of tacit as well as explicit knowledge. The domain of decision making still lies with the clinician and the patient, with the computer many years away from actually making decisions rather than supporting them. Finally, this perspective gives a new view on clinical governance, as it is basically the 'measurement' function of knowledge management.

# So that's the theory, what about the practice?

The following sections are a brief description of how the clinical computer is changing to become a partner in the consultation and a facilitator to knowledge management (both explicit and tacit).

## Using a computer as a partner in the consultation room

Clinical software, citizens' health consumerism, clinician attitudes, clinician computer skills and organisational views are all changing. There have been predictions[11,13] of a new consultation model that incorporates both the patient and clinical computer as partners. This model needs to recognise the change in clinical method and attitudes as well as consultation dynamics. Resources such as the *Using the Computer in the Consulting Room* CD-ROM[14] will help clinicians adapt to the style, but clinical systems also need to change to:

- ease the load of data entry into the record
- support shared decision making between clinician and patient
- improve support for explicit knowledge management
- enable contextually relevant tacit knowledge management (e.g. e-communities of practice).

### PRODIGY *as a knowledge management program*

PRODIGY is a computerised knowledge base incorporating around 120 sets of clinical guidance that has been rigorously constructed. A software specification is available for the clinical software suppliers to integrate it into their patient records. It is also an educational outreach and marketing program that enables local networks of people to be built around a primary care organisation (PCO) supported by a national network of resource kits and other facilitators. However, it is also developing a community of practice support electronically to enable individual clinicians as well as facilitators to engage in the PRODIGY program. It can be envisaged that clinicians could develop specific discussions around the management of an individual patient within the context of PRODIGY guidance and/or the guidance itself, which could involve the author of the guidance.

## Some final thoughts

This chapter has highlighted the fact that health informatics covers a much broader area than just computers. It has developed a discussion of the role of health informatics in e-clinical governance and shown that converting data into information and knowledge is a complex problem that involves many changes, of which those related to computing are small compared to the human and organisational issues. It has sketched out a high-level view of how health informatics can help us move forward and in particular presents a model of knowledge management.

## References

1  Waring N (2000) To what extent are practices 'paperless' and what are the constraints to them becoming more so? *Br J Gen Pract* **50**: 46–7.
2  Fogarty L, Cundy P and Hassey A (1999) *Good Practice Guidelines for General Practice Electronic Patient Records.* Joint Computer Group of BMA and RCGP, London.

3  Komaroff AL (1979) The variability and inaccuracy of medical data. *Proc IEEE* **67**: 1196–207.

4  Koran LM (1975) The reliability of clinical methods, data and judgements. *N Engl J Med* **293**: 642–6, 695–701.

5  Kay S and Purves IN (1996) Medical records and other stories: a narratological framework. *Methods Inf Med* **35**: 72–88.

6  Brody H (1994) 'My story is broken; can you help me fix it?' Medical ethics and the joint construction of narrative. *Lit Med* **13**: 79–92.

7  Rector AL, Nowlan WA and Kay S (1991) Foundations for an electronic medical record. *Methods Inf Med* **30**: 179–86.

8  Purves IN (1993) The current state and future needs of the electronic medical record for primary healthcare: a pragmatic view for the United Kingdom. In: S Teasdale and P Bradley (eds) *Proceedings of the Annual Conference of the Primary Heath Care Specialist Group of the British Computer Society.* Primary Health Care Specialist Group, Worcester, pp 113–22.

9  Burnum JF (1989) The misinformation era: the fall of the medical record. *Ann Intern Med* **110**: 482–4.

10 Eddy DM (1990) Clinical decision making: from theory to practice. The challenge. *JAMA* **263**: 287–90.

11 Purves IN (1996) Facing future challenges in general practice: a clinical method with computer support. *Family Practice* **13**: 536–43.

12 Nonaka I and Takeuchi H (1995) *The Knowledge Creating Company.* Oxford University Press, Oxford.

13 Purves IN (1998) The changing consultation. In: J Harrison and T van Zwanenberg (eds) *GP Tomorrow.* Radcliffe Medical Press, Oxford, pp 31–49.

14 SCHIN (2001) *Using the Computer in the Consulting Room.* SCHIN, Newcastle.

# Further reading

Purves IN (1996) The paperless general practice: it is coming, but needs more professional input. *Br Med J* **312**: 1112–13.

Purves IN (1998) *The 1996 GP Computer Survey.* NHS Executive, Leeds.

# 3

# Concepts in clinical governance

*Louise Simpson*

---

**Key points covered in this chapter**

- An overview of clinical governance
- Delve deeper into some of the concepts behind clinical governance
- Look at the concepts of organisational learning and teamwork
- Review a template for assessing clinical governance capacity in organisations
- Clarify our knowledge and understanding of clinical governance

---

## Where did clinical governance come from?

Clinical governance has evolved since its introduction in the NHS White Paper. If we were to ask any PCG/T group for a definition of clinical governance we would get as many definitions as there were people in the room.

The classic definition of clinical governance is:

*A framework through which NHS organizations are accountable for continuously improving the quality of their services and safeguarding high standards of care by creating an environment in which excellence in clinical care will flourish.*[1]

In other words, clinical governance means developing a structured system so that looking at the quality of care is an everyday part of life in a GP practice. Quality is important to most people working in primary care and clinical governance can help demonstrate – and improve – that excellence. Clinical governance is about changing the way people work, demonstrating that leadership, teamwork and communication are as important to high-quality care as risk management and clinical effectiveness. Indeed, it is in the nature of clinical governance as a 'whole system' response to improving healthcare quality that it finds its power. A number of different approaches are pursued in patient care and Tim van Zwanenberg and Jamie Harrison's excellent book *Clinical Governance in Primary Care*[2] gives a few.

To summarise what is necessarily a complex overall concept – as an explicit whole-system response to quality – clinical governance embraces the following concepts:

- improving patient care
- implementing evidence-based medicine into everyday patient care
- clinical audit and reflection on individual and teamwork
- ensuring patient safety
- the management of risk
- lifelong learning and personal development
- getting the culture right – through leadership, teamwork and communication.

As we saw in Chapter 1, the implementation of clinical governance is tied closely to organisational learning and teamwork.

## Organisational learning and the learning organisation

Organisational learning occurs when there is a balance between culture, technology, communication, infrastructure and organisational structure.[3]

Organisations are collections of individuals brought together to achieve an explicit or implicit aim. Individuals' behaviour aggregates to organisational behaviour, but it does not follow that individual learning aggregates to organisational learning. This is an important point for clinical governance, where the success of the organisation is dependent on individual contributions. Harvey and Denton support this, saying that 'becoming a learning organisation is perceived as one way of reducing the cost of knowledge-acquisition'.[4] Sharing knowledge becomes as important as acquiring it in clinical governance (*see* Figure 3.1).

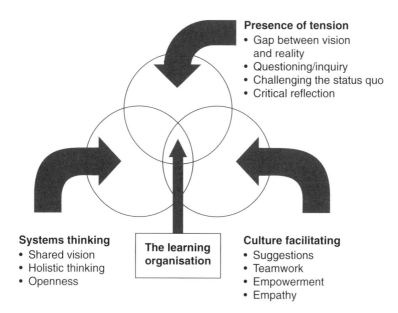

**Figure 3.1** The characteristics of learning organisations. Adapted from Luthans.[5]

# General practice with a memory?

Primary care practices, groups and trusts can achieve learning organisation status by establishing an organisational structure that supports open communication (inter-organisational as well as intra-organisational) along with a culture that values and enables learning (asking 'What went wrong?' not 'Who went wrong?' is an important approach if the blame culture is to be de-escalated here). This can be facilitated by a technological infrastructure that allows knowledge of good and bad practice to be accessed and utilised by team members. Access to quality (reliable, accurate, relevant and timely) information is essential in the development of the learning organisation, and the technology infrastructure will be essential in delivering this agenda. The threat is from information overload and 'knowledge underload' as portals open up easy, desktop access to an explosion of information resources of varying (and sometimes dubious) quality and efficacy.

# Learning lessons from secondary care

It is useful for us to look at the experiences of implementing clinical governance in secondary care. An assessment of secondary care trusts, carried out in 1999, aimed to establish a baseline of clinical governance capability and capacity. The assessment reviewed:

- What are the strengths and weaknesses in relation to current performance on quality?
- Which services and relationships may be problematic?
- To what extent is data collection in place for quality surveillance?
- Are there deficits in key mechanisms (e.g. for risk management)?
- How can explicit links be established between health improvement programmes, national service frameworks, etc?
- How should underpinning strategies (e.g. IM&T) be designed to support clinical governance in the organisation?

This gives us a useful and practical template for looking at the capacities of our own primary care organisations in introducing clinical governance, at both practice and PCG/T level. Importantly, it also recognises that clinical governance does not happen in isolation – in the words of Professor Aidan Halligan, the Director of Clinical Governance for the NHS, 'being explicit about quality' also means having the means to demonstrate excellent practice. Informatics is a means to that end.

The following points will help you to consider the impact of successfully implementing clinical governance:

- transforming organisational culture
- providing management and clinical decision support systems
- ensuring effective professional development
- establishing a flow of timely valid information on quality
- recognising, valuing and developing the excellence of NHS staff
- encouraging and developing leaders to inspire the culture change.[6]

Some simple questions about clinical governance practice are a good starting point in helping to both understand the concepts behind clinical governance and provide a guide for implementing the necessary cultural change (*see* Box 3.1).

---

**Box 3.1  Six key questions to reflect on clinical governance practice[7]**

- Do I reflect on my practice (perhaps with a clinical supervisor)?
- Am I using the most up-to-date evidence to influence the care I give?
- Am I involved in auditing the care the patients receive?
- Am I involving my patients in their care planning and delivery?
- Am I confident about raising concerns about patient care?
- Is my personal development plan based on service need as well as personal aspirations?

---

Phipps' points are particularly useful because their focus is on the individual and his or her relationships, emphasising that clinical governance is the responsibility of everyone *in* the team and not an external factor.

Quality is now a statutory obligation for NHS clinical organisations, but it is important to recognise that it involves *everyone* in the team, not just those with 'clinical governance' in their job title. It also requires the skills and expertise of all the team to succeed. If the byword of clinical governance is 'quality', then informatics can and should play a key role in 'doing the right thing, first time, every time'.

# References

1   Scally G and Donaldson LJ (1998) Clinical governance and the drive for quality in the new NHS in England. *Br Med J* **317**: 61–5.
2   van Zwanenberg T and Harrison J (2000) *Clinical Governance in Primary Care.* Radcliffe Medical Press, Oxford.
3   Stonehouse G and Pemberton J (1999) Learning and knowledge management in the intelligent organisation. *J Participation and Empowerment* **7**(5).
4   Harvey C and Denton J (1999) To come of age: the antecedents of organisational learning. *J Management Studies* **36**(7).
5   Luthans F (1998) *Organisational Behaviour.* McGraw-Hill, New York.
6   Donaldson LJ (2000) Clinical governance: a mission to improve. *Br J Clin Governance* **5**(1): 6–8.
7   Phipps K (2000) Viewpoint. *Br J Clin Governance* **5**(2): 69–70.

# 4

# Doing what we already do

*Paul Robinson*

---

**Key points covered in this chapter**

- Doing what we already do – patient care

- Using the computer in the consulting room with the patient, before the patient enters the room and after the patient has left (in between patients)

- Patient involvement

- The 'triadic' relationship and the 'new' consultation (partnership over paternalism)

- Lifelong learning

- Personal development programmes

---

This chapter deals with some practical aspects of bringing e-clinical governance into the life and work of practitioners. The purpose of healthcare is to provide the best for the patient, and the purpose of clinical governance is to help the practitioner provide that. Whatever the quality of the information and however slick the information technology, it will only help the patient or the doctor if they take it on board and incorporate it into their thoughts and actions. For both doctor and patient this represents a learning activity, and the human aspects of the communication are at least as important as the electronic.

In this chapter, we will consider four apparent contradictions.

- Paying attention to the patient: using the computer in the consultation.
- Medical knowledge as the practitioner's experience: medical knowledge as science.
- Involving the patient on equal terms: medical power and medical knowledge.
- Learning about what interests you: learning in areas of uncertainty.

It is easy, perhaps customary, to portray these pairings as opposites. The purpose of this chapter is to show how e-clinical governance can bring these contradictions together and will show how these opposites can attract.

## Using the computer in the consulting room

In general practice, the consultation is the key encounter and the consulting room is the forum in which most of these encounters occur. GPs are spending more and more time in their consulting rooms. This is because surgery appointments are increasing in number, while home visits are declining, and also because the consulting room is the place where the GP's computer sits. GPs use their computers in between surgeries and in between patients: sometimes for recording information, sometimes for communication, sometimes for learning.

We'll look at the use of the computer outside the consultation later, but first we need to tackle the thorny issue of using the computer during the consultation. Although it was shown that use of the keyboard and mouse could be 'backgrounded', so that it does not interfere with the inter-personal processes of the consultation, many GPs are concerned that using the computer during the course of the consultation may impair the rapport between doctor and patient.

## Rapport improves clinical outcomes

It is well known that rapport improves clinical outcomes. This is not just to say that you feel better after sharing rapport with another person. Studies of conditions such as respiratory infections and chronic headache show that the key variable in how quickly the patient recovers is not whether a prescription is offered, what prescription is offered or the seniority of the practitioner: it is whether or not the patient felt the practitioner understood his or her concerns about the condition. The same effect may be framed in terms of the doctor–patient relationship or the placebo effect: things that all experienced GPs understand intuitively and value.

Further, clinicians learn at an early stage in their careers that it is not 'cool' to take notes in front of the patient. As a young medical student, just let loose on the wards, the future GP has to concentrate so hard on getting right the catechism of questions that elicit early 'histories' that he or she has to write the answers down or they would be forgotten. One of the badges of the experienced houseman is the ability to manage the clinical encounter and then sit at the ward station writing up the case notes and ordering observations, tests and medication. Such lessons, hard learnt, are difficult to forget and GPs who are extremely skilled at computer use will shy away from using the keyboard while the patient is with them.

Third, there are concerns about dividing attention between the computer screen and the other person in the room. The human brain may be viewed as an extremely rich and complex network. However, it is *one* network and it seems that one network means one consciousness. We cannot attend to two things at the same time: if our attention is fully engaged on one narrative we cannot attend to another narrative at the same time.

Finally, we know that patients often say something important after a break in the dialogue. This is what lies behind the deliberate use of silence in some consultations. It also explains the well-known 'By the way doctor . . .' from the patient, hand on door handle, that heralds the most important reason for attending.

Against this, clinical governance is one of the drivers encouraging use of the computer during the consultation. Most GPs generate prescriptions on the computer at the end of the consultation, but the effective use of electronic records, templates, guidelines, information sources and on-line decision support will all require the practitioner to attend to, and interact with, the computer while the patient is in the room. How can this be done without throwing the baby (rapport) out with the bathwater?

## Information in the consulting room

A group at SCHIN has been looking at videotapes of GPs using the computer while consulting. Preliminary results show that it *is* possible to attend to the computer and the patient in the same consultation, but not at the same time. This can be done without damaging the inter-personal quality of the consultation.

The trick is to control the structure and sequence of the consultation, or make use of the structure that emerges, so that the practitioner does not have to try to divide his or her attention. Different GPs use different strategies and different skills to do this; the important thing is that it can be done, and the skills required are skills that can be taught.

The other thing that we have seen in this research is failure to pick up messages from the patient. This usually happens when the GP is engaged in an interactive task, such as generating a prescription. The special skills that can be taught also need to be learnt and rehearsed.

What is emerging from this research is a way of bringing together the first pair of contradictions mentioned at the start of the chapter. Instead of *either* using the computer *or* maintaining rapport, it is using the computer *and* maintaining rapport. What is also emerging is that there is a wide variation between GPs in how much they are prepared to share with the patient, in terms of sharing access to the screen, sharing information, sharing control of the interaction and sharing themselves. We will return to this later in the chapter.

Four key things to consider about using the computer in the consulting room are:

- Exploit – or manage – the structure of the consultation so you don't have to do two things at once.
- Pick up cues and messages from the patient.
- Share access to the screen, share access to information and share control of the interaction with the patient.
- Think about how your desk layout impacts on the dynamic.

## When the patient is not present

So far we have established that it is possible to make full use of the computer during the consultation and not lose out on the person-to-person interaction. There may, of course, be good reasons why the practitioner may choose not to use the computer as an information source during the consultation, including reasons of time and uncertainty. If you are not sure what you are looking for, searching can be time-consuming (*see* Chapters 5 and 6 for more on this). The GP may be uncertain of his or her own IT skills, or unsure of the content or format of what he or she is going to find. It is disturbing to have your own ideas contradicted or challenged and handling that is hard enough, but what if the information you retrieve from the computer system, or the Internet, is bad news for the patient? It is important to be explicit about these issues, especially if persuading a colleague to start to use the computer for the first time, and also to recognise there are strategies for managing the dissonance.

# Some ideas from the theory of learning

## How much information can you handle?

First, there is a limit to the amount of information that a person (patient or practitioner) can handle at any one time. It has also been shown in studies of the effect of patient education in people with chronic disorders that success depends on providing timely information, appropriate to the person's emotional and physical trajectory throughout the condition. If you think you are overloading the patient with information, or that there is stuff that they should know but are not quite ready for, it may be best to break off at that point. Rather than give out a leaflet when the patient is already 'full', it may be better to use some time before the next consultation to find some material appropriate to that individual, and use that material to organise the next bit of information giving.

## Reflection

Reflection is a key part of the learning process. Some writers, including Kolb,[1] think that learning cannot take place without reflection. Schon[2] has described the way that experts can reflect in action (i.e. think about what they are doing while they are doing it), and experienced GPs are able to do this in the consultation. However, the consultation is a very busy activity. A lot happens, so there is a lot to reflect on. For this reason, issues that deserve reflection may emerge a little after the event (between patients) or later on (between surgeries). The computer as information source can be used at these different times, and the computer systems should support this deferred learning.

## That uncomfortable feeling . . .

Learning relies on 'cognitive dissonance'. Cognitive dissonance is a term used for the discomfort felt when a person is exposed to information that conflicts with their previously held views. It is an emotional discomfort and can lead the individual to dismiss either the message or messenger without further thought. On the other hand, the new information may be accepted uncritically. More often, the discomfort is resolved by seeking information from other sources to corroborate or refute the new idea. This conflict may be 'chewed over' for some time before the corroboration is sought and that is another reason why the practitioner may look for information outside the consultation.

We need to remember that it is not just the GP, nurse or other clinician who is interested in learning about health, and it is not only the GP who has access to electronic health information. Domestic use of computers is increasing at least as fast as professional use. We could have written a section with the title 'Using the computer when the doctor is not present'.

# Involving the patient

So far, we have dealt with process aspects of how the presence of the computer may impinge on the doctor–patient relationship, and we have explored some of the circumstances in which the doctor and patient may use the computer as an information source. In this section we consider the computer, and the knowledge that it represents, as a participant in the consultation. The term 'the triadic consultation' has been coined to represent this idea. Here we are dealing with flows of information and knowledge, and the way these flows interact with power and identity within the consultation, and outside it.

# Science and experience/research and practice

Let us consider two of the contradictions further.

- Medical knowledge as the practitioner's experience: medical knowledge as science.
- Involving the patient on equal terms: medical power and medical knowledge.

The first of these reflects a broader distinction between knowledge as something created inside a person's head and knowledge as something external that is there to be discovered. Kolb[1] and other people who describe experiential learning consider the act of learning to be the process of actively creating knowledge inside the learner's brain. Knowledge of this kind is highly contextualised by personal, social and historical factors. It is the stuff of an individual's experience and expertise.

By contrast, scientific knowledge – the results of clinical trials and experiments – is thought of as being independent of personal context: it is 'objective' and generalisable to different people in different circumstances. Can these views of knowledge, or these types of knowledge, be brought together or are they irreconcilable opposites? Can medical knowledge be described as the person's experience (i.e. patient as well as practitioner)?

There has been much discussion about the gap between research and practice. The evidence-based medicine movement represents one attempt to close it. Narrative-based medicine, quality initiatives and clinical audit are others, and now clinical governance. Can e-clinical governance, by bringing evidence-based clinical guidance into the consultation through the use of informatics (including templates, protocols and decision support), move this quest forward? It depends.

Studies of professional expertise often use medical experts as their subjects. Expert behaviour is seen as being scripted; the sources of these scripts are mental schemata, which have a narrative structure and which embody the individual's experience. The key then is to incorporate the results of clinical trials, or the guidance based on them, into the clinician's schemata. Again that sentence should be rephrased. The patient is an expert in his or her own life and the guidance (or its consequences) has to become incorporated into his or her schemata as well as the clinician's.

In the past, doctors learnt about medical science in the medical school, the postgraduate centre or from books and journals. As well as the physical separation from the consulting room, this paradigm of transmission of medical knowledge contains a more powerful metaphor. This is that medical knowledge is for doctors to assimilate and then dispense. In social terms, this concentrates authority and power, and makes the doctor–patient encounter an unequal one. In educational terms, it is pedagogy rather than adult learning. Herein lies the problem: there is strong evidence that the adult learning model is the more effective, especially if the goal is to alter behaviour.

## Sharing the screen, hogging the keyboard

This brings us back to the research on GPs using the computer in the consultation, and the various degrees of sharing they displayed. It is possible to use timely, context-sensitive information in the consulting room in the old paradigm. The practitioner finds out the information, assimilates it and then dispenses the new-found wisdom to the patient. From what we have seen so far, the effect of this may be limited. How much more effective to involve the patient, not only by sharing the ability to see the computer screen, but also by taking account of their needs in deciding what information to seek, perhaps even to use the keyboard or mouse.

## Extelligence

So how does this help us resolve those two contradictions? As far as the two types of knowledge are concerned, e-clinical governance offers the opportunity to incorporate external knowledge (represented by clinical knowledge, guidance and so on, embodied in the system) into everyday practice, and so into the schemata of doctor and patient. It allows the science to become part of their experience. More subtly, the act of seeking information becomes a part of accepted practice: enquiry becomes part of the schemata of doctor and patient.

Stewart and Cohen[3] have coined the term 'extelligence' for knowledge and tools that are outside people's heads. Here we are talking about extelligence in the consultation, and the way the computer can bring vast amounts of extelligence into the consulting room.

By situating 'medical knowledge' in a box within the consulting room, but outside the human participants, the triadic consultation model can facilitate the development of a more equal relationship between practitioner and patient. 'The information is available here, let's find it out together.' The doctor's role changes from fount of knowledge to facilitator of learning.

There is an assumption at play here. For centuries, medical practitioners worked without scientifically proved treatments and relied almost entirely on the doctor–patient relationship. This strong relationship, with the placebo effect and pronoia* as its handmaidens, worked wonders. The placebo effect remains the most powerful of interventions. No one knows for sure whether a rigorous application of evidence-based guidelines, with no gap between research and practice, will serve us any better.

## Lifelong learning

We have explored e-clinical governance in educational terms, and considered how doctor and patient can learn separately and together from the electronic information system: within the consultation and outside it. In this last section, we will consider lifelong learning, from the professional's

---

* Pronoia is the opposite of paranoia, i.e. it is the deluded belief that everyone thinks you are wonderful. It is a concept that is particularly relevant to the doctor–patient interaction.

viewpoint. We will think about the fourth contradiction, the tendency of people to learn about what is interesting and safe rather than what is uncertain and risky (in terms of showing ignorance). Can e-clinical governance help resolve this contradiction?

The theory of adult learning says that learning is most effective when the learner perceives the topic to be relevant and interesting. Consequently, effective learning must meet the learner's felt needs. On the other hand, part of the agenda of clinical governance, and of the broader health service, is for practitioners to learn things that are relevant to the needs of the service and of patients. This is 'service-led' education. We know that doctors, and other professionals, tend to avoid learning about subjects for which they have a 'blind spot', or about which they feel uncomfortable but don't wish to declare as learning needs. This is just the territory where the 'real' needs of service-led education are likely to lie. Can 'real' needs and 'felt' needs be brought together?

## How do appraisal and mentoring fit in?

One way to tackle this issue is by educational mentoring or appraisal. Different people understand different and overlapping things by these terms. 'Mentor' carries connotations of a less directive, facilitative and developmental role, while 'appraiser' fits more with ideas of management and control. Appraisal can be formative too. The basic process of appraisal is for the practitioner to spend some time reflecting on his or her practice. This time is used to prepare a written submission, which is passed to the appraiser before the appraisal interview and then used as the basis of the interview. By framing the process of reflection in the context of established national and local priorities, and by using some of the tools of clinical governance (such as audit, significant event reviews, performance data) the practitioner can situate his or her performance within the needs of the service. The act of relating this story to the appraiser helps the practitioner to appreciate the 'real' needs and so incorporate them into the subjective 'felt' needs. The needs can then be turned into a learning plan. As with the conflicting views of knowledge discussed earlier, what this process is doing is bringing the external definitions into the person's subjective arena.

# IT and the 'e' in e-clinical governance

How do IT and informatics help here? First, audit and the collection and interpretation of performance data are much easier done with electronic IT. Second, the process of appraisal (for both appraiser and practitioner) can be supported and facilitated by electronic media such as the NHS Appraisal Toolkit (www.appraisals.nhs.uk). Third, this appraisal toolkit can be available as an information source and decision support during the appraisal interview. This models the triadic consultation, and if used skilfully will have the same benefits on learning and on issues of power and ownership.

# Some final thoughts

This chapter has looked at practical aspects of how the computer on the practitioner's desk can situate clinical governance within the consulting room and within the consultation. We have highlighted four pairs of apparent contradictions, and shown how these contradictions can be resolved. Behind these contradictions lie the essence and purpose of clinical governance. Adding the 'e' to e-clinical governance has two effects. One is to support what we are already doing. In that respect it is not about doing new things, more a new way of doing the same things. The other effect is to help resolve these contradictions in ways that paper-based methods do not, and cannot. Partnership and information sharing at last become possible.

# References

1   Kolb D (1984) *Experiential Learning*. Prentice Hall, Englewood Cliffs, NJ.
2   Schon D (1983) *The Reflective Practitioner: how professionals think in action*. Maurice Temple Smith, London.
3   Stewart I and Cohen J (1997) *Figments of Reality: the evolution of the curious mind*. Cambridge University Press, Cambridge, pp 243–70.

# Further reading

Dowie J (1996) The research practice gap and the role of decision analysis in closing it. *Health Care Anal* **4**: 1–14.

Greatbach D, Luff P, Heath C and Campion P (1993) Interpersonal communication and human–computer interaction: an examination of the use of computers in medical consultations. *Interacting with Computers* **5**: 193–216.

Kay S and Purves IN (1996) Medical records and other stories: a narratological framework. *Methods Inf Med* **35**: 72–88.

Robinson PJ and Heywood P (2000) What do GPs need to know? The use of knowledge in general practice consultations. *Br J Gen Pract* **50**: 56–9.

www.schin.ncl.ac.uk/iiCR/

# 5

# Evidence-based medicine

*Helen Raison*

---

**Key points covered in this chapter**

- What is evidence-based medicine or EBM?

- The 'process' of EBM

- e-Literature searching – what's out there on-line

- Other e-sources and key clinical journals

- e-Critical appraisal

- NHS initiatives around EBM

- e-Tools to help with EBM in the consultation

---

This chapter introduces the concept and process of 'evidence-based medicine' (EBM) and gives advice on electronic sources of evidence and critical appraisal. It also introduces some of the new NHS initiatives that are related to quality, clinical governance and EBM, and briefly covers some health informatics solutions, such as computerised clinical decision support systems.

# What is evidence-based medicine or EBM?

Evidence-based medicine can be thought of as the integration of best research evidence with clinical expertise and patient values.

EBM may seem more worthwhile if you view it in practical terms. It is a way of making sure patients get the *best management* of their disease, which will ensure they recover in the minimum amount of time and return to the most fit they can be. This is most likely to happen if the patient is managed by a well-informed primary care team that has not had to see the patient a number of times because the first treatments they tried did not work. It is highly likely that some of the treatments we think are the best are, in fact, not as effective as our medical training led us to believe. This is summed up in the words of Dr Sydney Burwell, Dean of Harvard Medical School:

> *My students are dismayed when I say to them that half of what you are taught as medical students will in 10 years have been shown to be wrong. The trouble is, none of your teachers know which half.*[1]

So if we accept that we may not know what the current best management is, even if we think we do, we know we have to find it. Finding the best management is about tapping into the research evidence, and then applying it to each patient. As there is so much evidence out there, it is an impossible task to know the latest information about everything. Instead, knowing where to look for the answers you need, and how to apply them in practice, is the key to surviving in an EBM world. GP computer systems, the Internet and other health informatics tools can make some of this process more manageable. This section will give you a brief overview of the EBM process, and some related issues, and point you towards some of the resources and health informatics solutions available to help you get to grips with EBM.

# The 'process' of EBM

The pure process of EBM is set out in Table 5.1, and it is good practice for everyone to understand these steps, even if there is no realistic chance of carrying them out on a regular basis. We have included some pointers about how to learn more about the process, but for those who will not be carrying out all the steps, valid 'shortcuts' are described later.

| Table 5.1 | The EBM process |
|---|---|
| *Stage in process* | *How can you practically achieve this?* |
| Step 1: Convert the need for information (about prevention, diagnosis, prognosis, therapy, causation, etc.) into an answerable question | This step is needed if you wish to personally define the search criteria you want to use in Medline or any other literature-searching tool. It is not a step practised commonly by most GPs, but is worth knowing about. If you want to know more the book *Evidence-based Medicine – how to teach and practice EBM*[1] is a good starting point. Librarians and clinical effectiveness centres should also be able to guide you to help |
| Step 2: Track down the best evidence with which to answer that question | This step involves doing a full literature search, and is often the step carried out by medical librarians, researchers or medical informatics specialists. Ideally we should all have skills in using search tools such as Medline, and they should be learned from those who literature search on a regular basis. If you want to know more about literature searching and retrieval, clinical effectiveness facilitators in PCGs, trust libraries, local interest groups or national EBM organisations will all be able to help you |
| | It is worth being aware of some of the more useful, comprehensive, good-quality sources of evidence, as you can access these without being accomplished at searching Medline. These sources do the hard work of searching, appraisal and synthesis for you. We cover some of these later in this chapter |
| Step 3: Critically appraise the evidence for its validity (closeness to the truth), impact (size of the effect) and applicability (usefulness to clinical practice) | Being able to look critically at a piece of research and work out if it is valid and whether its findings are significant and applicable to patients is a very valuable skill |
| | Critical appraisal skills are usually practised by professionals working in clinical governance, EBM and quality assurance. They are also a skill of many public health professionals. If you want to improve your own critical appraisals skills there are local and national courses, Internet sites and books to help you.[2] We cover some of these later in this chapter |
| Step 4: Integrate the critical appraisal with our clinical expertise, and with our patient's unique biology, values and circumstances | This takes practice, and group sessions within the PCG are a useful way of discussing how best to change to an evidence-based approach. Many national guidelines and policies, such as the National Service Frameworks, give some advice on how to integrate evidence into practice. Decision support systems used in primary care, such as PRODIGY, are designed to integrate EBM with patient characteristics. PRODIGY is described later |
| Step 5: Evaluate our effectiveness and efficiency in executing steps 1–4 and seek ways to improve them both for next time | Self-evaluation in its widest context is a key part of clinical governance. Performance against set criteria is part of clinical audit. Sometimes it is easier to use a group to evaluate your effectiveness at EBM, for example at a general practice surgery meeting |

The following sections will guide you to some of the resources for each EBM step. Many of these resources are available over the Internet. The Internet has been the single biggest advance that has improved access to information, including evidence. But beware! Information overload can be as much of a threat as poor information access, and poor information quality.

The World Wide Web (WWW) is easy to use, and even those not familiar with computers find that, with a little training, the Web offers a huge opportunity to access knowledge that used to take weeks or months to get hold of. Health informatics solutions such as clinical decision support systems or EBM organisations such as the National Institute for Clinical Excellence (NICE) are designed to perform many of the EBM process steps for you, and can also be accessed via the Web. They are discussed later in the chapter.

# e-Literature searching

## Carrying out an e-search

The most commonly used medical literature database is Medline. As well as being the largest, it was also the first one available for electronic searching. It can be accessed through the Internet. The number of ways of accessing a Medline service is growing, and many of them are free. Two of the most common routes are via PubMed and the BMA.

- Medline (via its makers, the US National Library of Medicine) www.ncbi.nlm.nih.gov/pubmed
- Medline (via the British Medical Association) www.bma.com
  *you can access Medline Plus via this website if you are a BMA member, but if you are not you can link to the US PubMed site as above.*

There are many other searchable databases, although they usually contain far fewer articles than Medline. Libraries in hospitals, universities and some in primary care will be able to direct you towards many of these.

There are also specialist evidence-based databases that are available online or on CD-ROM. These databases contain only research that has already been critically appraised, or has been carried out following very specific methodologies. For example:

- The Cochrane Library      www.cochrane.org
  *NB: access to Cochrane is by subscription*

- Best Evidence/Evidence Based      www.bmjpg.com
  Medicine

## Other e-sources of evidence

Instead of trawling through databases, it is often possible to identify the research centre that did the work or the journal in which the work was published. In these cases, it is often quicker to go straight to the journal, organisation or report you are after. Most major research centres publish in journals, many of which are electronic and available on the Web. Drug companies also report in journals, and in the commercial domain, but this research must always be read taking into account that often it has been published because it is positive and might not have been published if it had been negative. The NHS Research and Development Programme (www.doh.gov.uk/research) funds relevant new primary care research and will be a source of future research findings. The National Research Register (www.update-software.com/National) is a database of ongoing and recently completed research projects funded by, or of interest to, the UK's NHS.

## Key clinical journals

There are thousands of medical journals; some of those that consistently publish good-quality research are listed below. Again, although they are all available in paper format they are usually accessible at their own websites.

- *British Medical Journal*      www.bmj.com
- *New England Journal of Medicine*      www.nejm.com
- *JAMA*      www.jama.ama-assn.org
- *The Lancet*      www.thelancet.com/journal
- *Annals of Internal Medicine*      www.annals.org/
- *Archives of Internal Medicine*      www. archinte.ama-assn.org

There are some websites via which a range of journals are available, for example Science Direct (publishers Elsevier Science at www.sciencedirect.com).

## Key EBM summary journals and books

A growing number of periodicals summarise the best evidence in traditional journals, making their selections according to explicit criteria for merit, providing structural abstracts of the best studies and also commenting on their clinical applicability. The most prolific and widely accepted of these are those published under the title *Evidence-Based . . .* and include *Evidence-Based Medicine, Evidence-Based Mental Health, Evidence-Based Nursing, Evidence-Based Health Care Policy and Practice* and *Evidence-Based Cardiovascular Medicine* (*see* www.ebm.bmjjournals.com).

There are also textbooks that integrate evidence-based information from a wide range of sources, and inevitably they are also available on the Web. *Clinical Evidence* is one of the best examples of such a book (*see* www.clinicalevidence.com).

# e-Critical appraisal

Once potentially useful articles have been identified through a literature search they need to be critically appraised. There are many poor-quality studies the results of which should be discounted, while the good-quality studies should be identified and their results used to improve clinical practice. Practising critical appraisal can be done almost completely by using checklists. Standard checklists will help to identify papers that are likely to contain useful evidence. Standard lists can usually be applied to any research paper, irrespective of the research method that was used. An example of a standard checklist is shown in Box 5.1.

---

**Box 5.1 A checklist for critically appraising published research**

- Are conflicts of interest declared?
- Are the aims clearly stated?
- Was the sample size justified?
- Are the measurements likely to be valid and reliable?
- Are the statistical methods described?
- If appropriate, were there controls, randomisation and double blinding?
- Did untoward events occur during the study?
- Were the basic data adequately described?
- Do the numbers add up?

- Was the statistical significance assessed?
- What do the main findings mean?
- How are null findings interpreted?
- Are important effects overlooked (e.g. safety)?
- How do the results compare with previous reports?
- What implications does the study have for your practice?

List adapted from *The Pocket Guide to Critical Appraisal.*[3]

Understanding how to use a checklist is the human skill of critical appraisal, and there are numerous ways of learning how to do this. Some electronic sources include the National electronic Library for Health (*see* www.nelh.nhs.uk) and the NHS Critical Appraisal Skills Programme or CASP (*see* www.casp.org.uk). Both websites give more information on critical appraisal and also details of workshops where these skills can be practised.

# NHS-based initiatives specialising in EBM: NICE, NeLH, NSFs

Not everyone has the skills, access to resources, time and money to follow the classic EBM process. In fact, even people who are keen on EBM have difficulty going through the process in the busy NHS environment. More important, perhaps, is that if everyone carried out their own EBM processes there would be a huge duplication of effort resulting in a waste of NHS time and money.

These limitations have been realised within the NHS, and a number of specialist organisations have been set up to help bring EBM to healthcare professionals (Table 5.2). Many of these produce summaries of evidence and guidelines.

Two such organisations are NICE and the National electronic Library for Health (NeLH). The National Service Frameworks (NSFs) also provide structured ways for working and draw on evidence-based medicine. The Department of Health in its paper on clinical governance recommends that health authorities, PCG/Ts and NHS trusts monitor their professional staff to ensure they are gaining access to such knowledge resources.[4] The expectation is that clinical standards set by NICE and the NSFs will be implemented nationwide, and that these standards will be monitored by the Commission for Health Improvement (CHI).

| **Table 5.2**   NHS-based initiatives specialising in EBM | |
|---|---|
| *Initiative* | *Website* |
| National Institute for Clinical Excellence: NICE is part of the NHS, and its role is to provide patients, health professionals and the public with authoritative, robust and reliable guidance on current 'best practice'. The guidance will cover both individual health technologies (including medicines, medical devices, diagnostic techniques, and procedures) and the clinical management of specific conditions | www.nice.org.uk |
| National Service Frameworks: NSFs set national standards and define service models for a specific service or care group, put in place programmes to support implementation and establish performance measures against which progress within an agreed timescale will be measured | www.doh.gov.uk/nsf/about.htm |
| National electronic Library for Health: the NeLH programme is working with NHS libraries to develop a digital library for NHS staff, patients and the public in order to provide access to information for all | www.nelh.nhs.uk |

The NHS also has a number of other evidence-based initiatives, including: centres that list ongoing research, such as the National Research Register; databases containing good-quality research findings, such as the Cochrane Library; and evidence-based decision support systems, such as PRODIGY (Table 5.3).

# Other evidence-based centres and groups and guideline producers

The Scottish Intercollegiate Guidelines Network (SIGN) publishes authoritative and useful guidelines on its website (*see* www.sign.ac.uk).

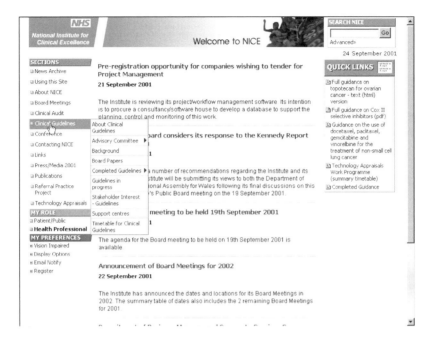

The NICE website.

The Centre for Evidence Based Medicine at the University of Oxford is one of the most well-established EBM centres in England (*see* www.cebm.jr2.ox.ac.uk).

Many professional organisations now focus on clinical governance and evidence-based medicine. Although too numerous to list, their websites give further information on how these are applied within the different specialities. The Royal College of General Practitioners publishes information and advice on quality and standards in primary care. These 'quality and standards' cover quality assessment for GPs, clinical governance and evidence-based healthcare (*see* www.rcgp.org.uk/rcgp/webmaster/quality_and_standards.asp). Regional groups can often provide a useful local focus, such as the Northern and Yorkshire Evidence-based Practice Group (www.eb-practice.fsnet.co.uk).

There are thousands of EBM websites on the WWW. 'Netting the Evidence' has been available for at least 5 years and is based at the University of Sheffield (*see* www.shef.ac.uk/~scharr/ir/netting/). It is updated by a professional with a lot of experience in EBM and is a worthwhile site to use as a starting place for accessing other evidence-based sites. The site also has a downloadable textbook: *The ScHARR Guide to Evidence-based Practice*. The well-known *Bandolier* is written by evidence experts based in Oxford (*see* www.jr2.ox.ac.uk/bandolier/).

| Table 5.3 Other NHS evidence-based initiatives | |
|---|---|
| *Initiative* | *Website* |
| The Cochrane Library | www.cochranelibrary.co.uk |
| The NHS Centre for Reviews and Dissemination: under the rearrangements of some organisations following recent government health White Papers, the Effective Health Care Bulletins have come under the auspices of NICE. This centre has produced a number of articles on evidence-based medicine which are worth a read; for example, *Getting Evidence Into Practice*[5] | www.york.ac.uk/inst/crd |
| PRODIGY: a decision support system for primary care developed for the NHS by the NHS. Under the rearrangements of some organisations following the recent government health White Papers, the clinical content of PRODIGY has come under the auspices of NICE | www.prodigy.nhs.uk |
| Chief Medical Officer: the CMO's department does not specialise in EBM, but has a broad interest in clinical governance and evidence-based practice and is a site worth book-marking on your computer | www.doh.gov.uk/cmo/cmo.htm |

Rather than providing access to a range of evidence sources, *Bandolier* does its own critical appraisal of research and then publishes them in a leaflet or on the Web. It is written in a very practical and friendly style and is a good way of keeping up to date with some aspects of EBM.

# e-Tools to help with EBM and clinical governance in the consultation

There are a range of electronic CD-ROMs, software programs, websites and decision support systems available to support healthcare workers today. A number of them have been specifically designed for use via the computer during a busy day, and some are integrated into the clinical system. Others are simply textbooks that have been transformed into electronic versions, but nonetheless these are still useful reference tools.

## CD-ROMs

CD-ROMs can be run on your computer. A wide range of healthcare titles is available, and many different publishers sell them or provide them free of charge. The challenge is separating the good- from the poor-quality CD-ROMs. Those available from authoritative sources are probably the most reliable and contain anything from summaries of the latest evidence to details of the drugs that can be prescribed in the UK, e.g. the electronic BNF (*British National Formulary*). The paper version of the *BNF* has been the prescribing reference book of choice for many decades. The *BNF*'s information has been based on sources such as experts and traditional literature reviews, but it is now adopting EBM practices and basing its information more and more on systematic reviews of the literature and critical appraisal of research reports. The CD-ROM is not yet as popular as the paper version but as its design improves and users become more computer literate, that may change. Much of the data in the *BNF* are drawn from the latest Summaries of Product Characteristics that the pharmaceutical companies provide on their drugs. These can also be accessed directly from the drug industry via the Internet at http://emc.vhn.net. The *BNF* is also available on the WWW to subscribers at www.bnf.org/BNFProductsFrame.htm.

## Computer-based decision support

Computerised decision support systems are designed to map complex clinical decision making to the supporting evidence. Many such systems have been focused on diagnosis, but more recently those that support patient management have received more interest. In the government's White Paper *Information for Health*,[6] management decision support systems such as PRODIGY are identified as one method of supporting healthcare workers in the NHS.

PRODIGY is a prescribing decision support system that is integrated into primary care computer systems. It contains evidence on around 120 conditions commonly encountered in general practice. The clinical evidence in the system is kept up to date by a team of doctors, pharmacists and research associates, and the updated information is issued approximately three times a year. Urgent information is issued immediately rather than waiting for the next issue date. PRODIGY adapts all the recommendations made by NICE, the NSFs and other evidence sources into useable electronic excerpts for primary care.

PRODIGY is more than an information-giving system, as it lists all the management options available for a condition and gives an indication of what the evidence is to support each option. For many conditions there are options for management interventions for which there is little or no evidence. These are still offered by the system. PRODIGY also contains patient information leaflets (the leaflet's information accurately reflects the evidence in language that most patients would be able to understand), and the system automatically generates prescriptions tailored to each patient. Referral information, investigation advice and follow-up pointers are all extras that are provided in the system, and are designed for use with the patient present in the consulting room. The system also automatically records relevant clinical terms (i.e. Read Codes) into the electronic patient record, thus ensuring the data collected on your patients are useful, detailed and consistent. PRODIGY is also available in its non-dynamic format on the website www.prodigy.nhs.uk. The information contained is identical to that contained in the decision support system, but the dynamic features (such as tailoring to the patient, printing of prescriptions and patient information leaflets) are not available and it should not be used for treating patients directly, but as a source of information.

PRODIGY is available from your computer supplier, who will arrange for it to be installed or activated on your practice system. For further information about PRODIGY you can contact the PRODIGY National Dissemination Office:

| PRODIGY Dissemination | Tel: 0191 243 6196 |
|---|---|
| National Office | Fax: 0191 243 6101 |
| Sowerby Centre (SCHIN) | Email: prodigy-enquiries@schin.ncl.ac.uk |
| University of Newcastle | |
| 16/17 Framlington Place | |
| Newcastle Upon Tyne | |
| NE2 4AB | |

Other e-tools are often made available via the individual suppliers of clinical systems to primary care. Details of these tools are available direct from the suppliers.

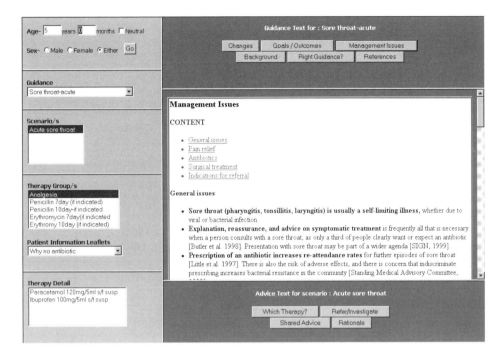

The PRODIGY decision support system.

## Some final thoughts

Evidence-based medicine will help to improve the quality of care in the NHS. The danger is that we will become swamped in a mountain of research findings and not be able to apply them to patients effectively. This is potentially compounded if there are conflicting sources of evidence that leave healthcare professionals wondering which source to believe. This is where informatics can help – enabling access to relevant EBM and clinical guidance at the crucial point.

The NHS initiatives such as NICE, NeLH, Prodigy and the concept of clinical governance offer structures, frameworks and resources for communicating evidence clearly, so that health professionals can continue to concentrate on treating patients while ensuring the best treatments are being offered.

## References

1　Sackett DL *et al.* (2000) *Evidence Based Medicine: how to practice and teach EBM* (2e). Churchill Livingstone, London.
2　Greenhalgh T (2000) *How to Read a Paper: the basics of evidence based medicine* (2e). BMJ Books, London.
3　Crombie DK (1996) *The Pocket Guide to Critical Appraisal.* BMJ Books, London.
4　NHS Executive (1999) *Clinical Governance: quality in the new NHS.* Department of Health, London.
5　Centre for Reviews and Dissemination (1999) Getting evidence into practice. *Effective Health Care Bulletin* **5**(1).
6　NHS Executive (1998) *Information for Health.* Department of Health, London.

# 6

# Risk management

*David Graham*

---

**Key points covered in this chapter**

- What is risk management?

- Where do we start?

- How can informatics help with risk management?

- A look at repeat prescribing

---

## What is risk management?

Whether we like it or not, the spiralling increase in medical litigation means complaints will have (or may already have had) an impact on every member of your primary healthcare team.

Statistics from the Medical Protection Society show that their members were 13 times more likely to be sued by patients in 1998 than in 1989. NHS figures show that the average rate of complaints is currently one per GP every year.

The litigious culture is not going to abate, especially when fanned by sensationalist journalism, adverts from opportunistic solicitors and the idea that there is a pot of gold at the end of every complaint. The effect of a complaint on a practitioner in terms of stress, damage to his or her reputation and future practice is considerable. Unless experienced first-hand, it is impossible to appreciate its impact.

The ideal solution is to avoid all complaints, which is clearly not possible given the nature of primary care unless you have a very reliable crystal ball or access to a time machine (please forward details to us if this is the case!). We therefore need to consider ways in which the risk of a complaint can be minimised. Experience in the US shows that while half of all successful medical negligence claims can be attributed to poor judgement on behalf of the doctor, the other half could probably have been avoided if appropriate risk management had been implemented. Bear in mind that, with respect to medical negligence, where the US leads, the UK follows.

## Where do we start?

The results of a survey published in 1998 by the Medical Defence Union (MDU) of the reasons for medical negligence claims over a 5-year period, revealed the causes to include:

- failure to diagnose or a delay in diagnosis: 51%
- medication errors: 26%
- management of pregnancy and labour: 7%
- other (administrative errors): 3%.

Clearly not all of these would have been influenced by risk management, but:

> A large number of these claims involve failures in systems which could be influenced by risk management techniques. For example, failure and delays in diagnosis could be avoided by introducing systems to ensure that test results are reviewed appropriately and patients are not lost to follow-up (MDU in 1998).

## How can informatics help with risk management?

Assuming that you are not now too depressed and are still reading, the purpose of this chapter is to consider some of the ways in which your electronic toolbag can be used to implement risk management. That big grey box of wires that sits on your desk, and seems to be linked to a television screen and a set of typewriter keys, is actually a wonderful tool for effecting risk management – if only you would turn it on and use it. We will consider some of the practical ways you can do this under the headings:

- Checks, warnings and system prompts.
- Pre-entered data.
- Organisation of data on the screen.
- The electronic patient record (EPR) summary screen.
- Computerised templates and protocols.
- Searches, audits and reports.

Please bear in mind that the following are only a few examples and suggestions designed to stimulate ideas at a practice/PCG/T level. It is important for every member to:

- identify risk
- assess the risk
- reduce or eliminate the risk
- constantly monitor your measures for controlling risk

in a way that is tailored to your own needs, and therefore initiate and maintain risk management as a tool that will become an integral part of practice life.

## *Checks, warnings and system prompts*

These are all risk management tools that can be used during the consultation. Your clinical computer system will already be set up to incorporate many of these. Some may pop up on the screen throughout the consultation. Examples include:

- Interactions between the drug that you are trying to prescribe and the repeat medication that you had forgotten your patient was taking.
- A screen to tell you that the systolic BP of 1400 that you are trying to enter is 'too high to be likely'.
- A reminder, when you are trying to prescribe amoxicillin, that you made an entry of 'penicillin allergy' in 1989.

You see, you are already using electronic risk management without realising it; that wasn't too painful, was it?

Other checks, warnings and system prompts can easily be set up on your system; indeed, they can be tailored to your individual practice needs. If nobody in the primary healthcare team (PHCT) has the skills to do this, contact your PCG/T who will be able to provide appropriate support. Examples include:

- A reminder that your patient is overdue a smear.
- A reminder that your patient has ischaemic heart disease (IHD), his last cholesterol level was 6.7 mmol/l and it has not been acted upon or rechecked.
- A warning that your patient had a splenectomy following a motorbike accident and does not seem to have received the recommended pneumococcal, Hib, influenza and meningococcal A & C vaccines.
- A prompt that the urine sample your patient has just handed in at reception has revealed glycosuria.
- A reminder that your patient with type 2 diabetes has not had his BP checked for 7 months.
- A reminder that your (otherwise well) patient with ear wax has not had her BP checked for 4 years.
- A prompt that the 17-month-old boy who has come for a review of his eczema has not received his MMR vaccination.

Checks, warnings and system prompts can be linked to prescriptions, whether acute or repeat. These can be considered in conjunction with the risk management of repeat prescribing described below. Examples include:

- A prompt that your patient with rheumatoid arthritis, whose repeat prescription for methotrexate you are about to sign, is overdue a check of her liver function tests.
- A warning that your patient with asthma is requesting his third salbutamol prescription in 4 days.
- A reminder that you have not checked the renal function of the patient with congestive cardiac failure, whose prescription for an ACE inhibitor you are about to sign.

## Pre-entered data

Some of the data included in your system software have the potential to be unhelpful and misleading, and therefore need consideration. Examples include the following.

- The prescription instruction 'as directed'; this is entirely meaningless, fraught with risk and should never be added to a prescription. The instruction to the patient should always be clear, e.g. take 4 times a day.
- Some instructions need to contain even more specific times, e.g. if a prescription for isosorbide mononitrate has the instruction 'take twice daily', this will probably eliminate the necessary nitrate-free interval; the prescription should read 'take twice daily, at 8 am and 2 pm'.

- Read codes such as 'BP control satisfactory' are unhelpful. Why should you be given the chance of adding such a vague comment when it is just as quick, and immeasurably more helpful, to record the BP exactly.

Such data will vary between systems. It is sensible to become aware of unhelpful pre-entered data as part of your own risk management, and therefore to avoid its use.

## Organisation of data on the screen

Each system supplier will set, as a default, the first screen to appear when a patient's record is accessed. This is usually the current screen. It can, however, easily be altered to show a prompt screen, a review screen or the medication screen. Again this is a personal choice.

Of far greater importance from a risk management viewpoint is the organisation of the patient's current screen. A current screen is just what it says; it should only contain current problems. Any dormant problems (or past problems that are no longer relevant) should be moved into the dormant screen. It is equally important to link problems under one title when appropriate, so that the screen is not cluttered with repeated entries of 'tonsillitis'. It is very relevant that your patient has attended every two months for the last six years with acute tonsillitis, but it is of far greater use if these entries are all under the same heading, rather than having 36 separate headings dominating a current screen.

The real danger of this is that the most important heading may be completely hidden several screens back. This may not seem too important as you may be absolutely certain that you know your patient well enough to be aware of his or her relevant history (surely an issue for risk management in itself!); but what about when you are away, and one of your partners (or even a locum) is struggling to deal with your dearest heartsink? The relevance of constipation as the eighth complaint on their list may be dismissed as unimportant, unless the entry of a right hemicolectomy four years ago for caecal carcinoma can easily be seen.

Although it may seem a daunting task to organise all the data, and keep them organised, the implications of not doing so are so great that you cannot ignore it for too much longer. One solution is to invest in some staff overtime to get the bulk of it done, and for all PHCT members to eat away at it continually.

## The EPR summary screen

All training practices have an obligation to provide summary cards in the patient records, and to keep them up to date. This is an excellent risk management tool which every practice should consider.

The move towards a paperless system means that summary cards will clearly need to become an integral part of the computerised record. The need to maintain this, update it and keep it relevant should be obvious to all (we hope), but again may seem a daunting task to initiate. As discussed above (Organisation of data), the longer you leave it, the longer you are ignoring a risk that may trip you up and land you in the proverbial! Again this may be an area where your PCG/T might consider providing some cash to employ a dedicated team or pay for some overtime to set this up. It is then up to you to maintain the summaries – this does not happen by magic.

## Computerised clinical guidelines, templates and protocols

We are all aware of the use of clinical guidelines. We are also all too aware of their limitations.

- We receive so many through the post and have so little time to read them.
- They seem to be out of date as soon as we start to use them, supplements and further updates arriving on the practice manager's desk at an increasing rate.
- It may be difficult to incorporate them effectively into our own practice.
- How many of us have time during a 10-minute (if you are lucky) consultation to dig out the appropriate protocol file and leaf through it until we find the section appropriate to the patient sitting opposite – it also gives the impression that we don't know what to do and are having to look it up in a manual!

Wouldn't it be a wonderful world if somebody could produce a set of computerised clinical guidelines, templates and protocols that:

- were automatically incorporated into our practice computer systems
- were updated and maintained so that we could concentrate on seeing patients
- were peer-reviewed and validated
- were easy to use by GPs and nursing staff
- would interact with the patient's computer record

- covered acute and chronic disease management
- would promote audit of every aspect of disease management
- would drastically reduce the chance of the wrong prescription being issued by mistake (e.g. it would be impossible to prescribe penicillamine accidentally while in the template for sore throat)
- provided education sections for the user
- provided patient information leaflets (we all know how little of the consultation is remembered by the patient after they leave)
- were free to the practice.

If such a system were available it would have an enormous impact on risk management for every user – each would surely pass 'the Bolam test' in law. The Bolam case held that a doctor is not in breach of the duty of care 'if he has acted in accordance with a practice accepted as proper by a responsible body of medical men skilled in that particular art'.

Such a system is available – PRODIGY provides all the features described above. You may be able to get it by simply contacting your GP clinical system supplier and requesting it. You may also be interested to check out the health informatics program for the coronary heart disease (HIP for CHD) NSF at www.hipforchd.org.uk .

## Searches, audits and reports

Those of us who are old enough to remember the Medical Audit Advisory Group (MAAG) and the Primary Care Audit Group (PCAG) are aware that audit has been an important part of primary care for many years – clinical governance cannot take the dubious responsibility for its existence.

The establishment and maintenance of an effective programme of searches, audits and reports is a vital part of risk management. It should also be able to demonstrate that practice has changed (hopefully improved) as a result. This programme should be in place at every level, from practice to PCG/T to health authority to Department of Health.

The programme is most likely to be used effectively when the areas it covers have been identified as a result of risk management, and are therefore of interest and importance to the PHCT concerned. If the programme is run on a paper system, it will be time-consuming and difficult to maintain. It is far more likely to succeed if it is incorporated into your computer system, thus becoming manageable within the workload and time constraints of primary care. Exceptions are significant event audit and adverse incident reporting. These are two very important risk management tools that are based on real cases and incidents (often single) that have occurred in your practice; they may therefore be better managed on a paper system.

The programme will be tailored to your individual practice and will follow the identification and assessment of risk. Examples include:

- Have all women had a smear who should have done?
- Have all the smear results been received within 4 weeks?
- Do all patients with chronic obstructive pulmonary disease (COPD) attend the clinic annually for spirometry?
- Does every patient with IHD take anti-platelet therapy?
- Have we received all of our lab results via computer pathology links?
- Has every lab result been acted upon appropriately and within a suitable timescale?

The list could be endless and is only intended to stimulate ideas in your own practice.

## A look at repeat prescribing

Repeat prescribing is an area that warrants special mention. It accounts for over two thirds of all GP prescriptions in the UK and four fifths of the total cost. A practice of 10,000 patients may issue 25,000 repeat prescriptions annually. The task of issuing, checking and signing is tedious and repetitive. How many of us have sat signing a huge pile of repeats with one hand, leafing through the day's lab results with the other, while talking to a patient on the phone. Add to that the fact that it is Monday morning, it is half-term and two of your partners are away, you have an urgent home visit to do but the reception staff won't let you out until you have signed all of your absent partners' repeats . . . It soon becomes obvious that the risks are increasing exponentially.

Bear in mind the facts that:

- The figures published by the MDU showed that 26% of settled claims were directly related to problems in prescribing, monitoring or administering medicines.
- GPs have a legal responsibility for any prescription they sign, regardless of whether it was generated by them or was one of their partners' repeats.
- Errors easily occur from telephone requests; how often are reception staff asked for 'some of me little white pills, please love', often by people on polypharmacy.
- It takes much less time to sign a prescription than to see a patient and review their long-term drug therapy. A full review, however, saves time in the long term as it includes all chronic disease management.

It soon becomes clear that repeat prescribing is a minefield of risks. Of all the causes of error, prescribing is one area that practices should be able to minimise. A risk management policy for repeat prescribing is vital, and it should be tailored to each individual practice. Chapter 7 looks at this in more detail.

## Some final thoughts

This chapter has looked at the basic principles of risk management, how it can easily and effectively be introduced, and how your computer system can integrate it into your practice.

Don't be afraid of risk management – look on it as a friend who is there to stop you stumbling up any sort of creek without a paddle. A small amount of time invested now will pay huge dividends in the future. Don't ignore it in the same way that you ignored the advice as a house officer that you should start to plan for retirement!

# 7

# Patient information and consumer health informatics

*Rob Wilson*

---

**Key points covered in this chapter**

- What is consumer health informatics?
- What is the case for consumer health informatics?
- What is the relationship between clinical governance and consumer health informatics?
- Models of clinical governance from a consumer perspective
- Bringing it together
- Sources of consumer health informatics information to support clinical governance

---

Patients are also citizens and consumers. Access to information resources has exploded with the widespread penetration of Internet access, and there is a whole industry targeting your patients with the aim of keeping them extremely well informed about the most common – and most rare – of conditions. This chapter describes the role of consumer health informatics in the support and delivery of clinical governance.

# What is consumer health informatics?

Consumer health informatics is a broad term. Eysenbach has defined it as:

> **Consumer health informatics** is the branch of medical **informatics** that analyses **consumers'** needs for information; studies and implements methods of making information accessible to **consumers**; and models and integrates **consumers'** preferences into medical information systems.[1]

# A bold claim?

Society has seen the rise of the patient as an active consumer rather than a passive recipient of healthcare. The challenge consumer health informatics aims to meet is bridging the gap between the healthcare offered by professionals and organisations and that which the patient wants. The term consumer health informatics can mean one of two things: the information systems designed for use by patients or the means of bringing together doctors and patients in a partnership in order to communicate effectively.

The provision of access to a patient's own health record information has been argued to be an ethical and quality of care imperative for the health service. Also consumer health informatics is claimed to represent an opportunity to enhance and support the existing treatment process. What is the evidence for these claims?

# What is the case for consumer health informatics?

Patients are the primary source of information in healthcare. Their explanations of their symptoms and the tests performed on them make up the bulk of data presented in the healthcare process through the gateway of primary care. Patient evidence is also the basis for the majority of actions by clinicians, and patients' decisions about treatment have a direct bearing on whether or not it is a success.

However, there appears to be evidence that some of the current approaches to care may not be effective. A good example of this is the recent Royal Pharmaceutical Society report on treatment concordance. One of the key pieces of evidence suggested that as few as half of patients with chronic disease take their medicines effectively (www.concordance.org). The report suggests that the current model of patient and doctor relationships may not be fulfilling patients' needs and that a new approach to shared decision making and negotiation may be needed, and may be supported by informatics.

One of the key targets of the NHS Plan is to facilitate patient access to records by 2004. Pilot studies of patients having access to their records are under way as part of the NHS Information Authority ERDIP programme and early indications are that these are generally successful. In response to a survey conducted in one pilot site, patients said they thought they should have access to their records and that they would like to control access to records. Earlier work has also demonstrated that patient access to records improves the quality of the information in the records. More advanced applications work on the premise that information can both be gathered directly from the patient (monitoring of their activities/ condition) and entered directly to a remote system that can then suggest subsequent amendments to a patient's treatment.

Consumer health informatics systems can also be a means of providing tailored information and alternative treatment options (as an alternative or supplement to pharmaceutical interventions or referral), and of gathering information from patients about attitudes, choices and satisfaction. All these are opportunities to improve care in a systematic way. Research conducted on oncology patients has shown that accessing records and information tailored using records improved outcomes. Patients reported that they had learnt something new, thought the information was relevant, used the computer again and showed their computer printouts to others.[2]

This all sounds fine but how does it apply to clinical governance?

## What is the relationship between clinical governance and consumer health informatics?

This section outlines the relationships between the two concepts in terms of the types of provision that can be facilitated for health consumers or patients. The opportunities for consumer health informatics to support clinical governance are threefold as Figure 7.1 shows.

Several well-established themes in social medical research support the need for clinical governance from this perspective. With the trend towards improvements in patient-focused care we can see from Table 7.1 how the types of provision might relate to these key themes.

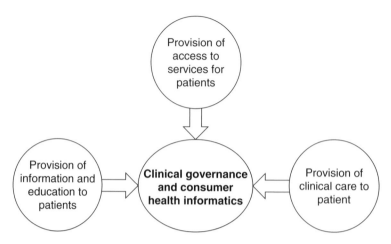

**Figure 7.1** Opportunities for consumer health informatics to support clinical governance.

Demonstrably improving the quality of care to patients in a consumer-centred way while improving the quality of relationships may seem like the holy grail of clinical governance: perfect yet unobtainable. Yet relatively simple changes to processes or policies can be put in place to improve the quality of care to patients. How can this be achieved?

**Table 7.1**   Some areas to address in health informatics

|  | *Quality of clinical care to patients* | *Quality of information and education to patients* | *Quality access to service provision for patients* |
|---|:---:|:---:|:---:|
| Shared decision making between clinicians and patients | ☺ | ☺ | |
| Knowledge transfer from clinicians to patients | ☺ | ☺ | |
| Compliance rates with treatment | ☺ | ☺ | |
| Patient general knowledge and recall | | ☺ | ☺ |
| Patient consultation and involvement in service development/delivery | | | ☺ |

Table 7.1 suggests areas to address in improving the quality of healthcare to consumers.

# Models of clinical governance from a consumer perspective

Clinical governance can support directly improved services at the one-to-one, one-to-many and many-to-many level. Figures 7.2 and 7.3 demonstrate ways of thinking about services that directly affect the experiences of consumers. The use of inconsistent terms is deliberate to show how 'consumers' may perceive common relationships.

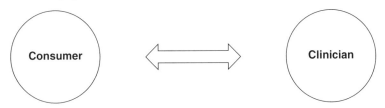

**Figure 7.2**   The one-to-one care process.

The sorts of care process that occur at a one-one level are usually those within the patient–clinician interaction. These are usually face-to-face interactions, but the use of simple devices such as telephones and email can change the nature of these interactions. Both the quality and process of these new forms of interaction can be supported using electronic means.

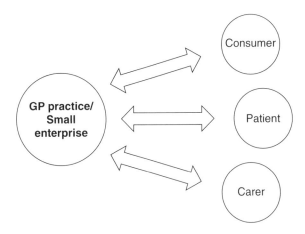

**Figure 7.3**   The one-to-many care process.

Two major points at which a clinical governance analysis could support the interaction between practices and individuals (one-to-many) are the scheduling of appointments and the organisation of repeat prescriptions. These are services that affect every consumer interacting with a practice (or small enterprise).

# The clinician–patient consultation and consumer health informatics tools (one-to-one)

At the individual level, an example of this could be the aim to increase the information available to patients. The first step should be to offer information about their condition to patients as a standard part of the consultation. A review of patient information leaflets has shown that information given in consultations has greater efficacy than that which is picked up in practice waiting rooms.[3] More and more information is becoming available to patients through a variety of sources. However, patients still value information from clinicians. An excellent source of information (including drawings and self-help group information) about common conditions and common scenarios in primary care are the patient information leaflets available in most GP software systems through the PRODIGY decision support system. These are written by GPs for use in consultations and are part of the EMIS system. They are also available through the Web on a number of sites (including www.prodigy.nhs.uk).

Six areas to reflect on for consultations might be:

- asking open questions
- fulfilling information needs
- checking patient's understanding
- involving patients in decision making and care planning
- seeking and recording informed consent
- being aware of local resources and support networks.

Other aspects of information sharing and using computers to support clinical care, including shared decision making, are explained elsewhere in Chapter 4 and outlined in *Using the Computer in the Consulting Room* CD-ROM available free of charge from the PRODIGY National Dissemination office.

# Consumer health informatics at an organisational level (one-to-many)

At the practice level, an example of where a clinical governance initiative can benefit from using a consumer informatics approach is repeat prescribing. The ordering and collection of repeat prescriptions is a common experience for most patients and their carers. Who are these patients?

## *The repeat prescribing experience*

Patients on repeat prescriptions, usually for a chronic condition, make up a high percentage of patients actively receiving care from a practice or primary care organisation. They usually are older, likely to be suffering from multiple health problems and represent those most likely to be referred to secondary care for specialist support. In short, these patients are the practice's most regular customers.

Figure 7.4 is adapted from the NHS Repeat Prescribing project report and shows the key points of the usual process of repeats. Practices can use the diagram to look at their repeat prescribing process and ask the following questions.

- Does the practice have a written repeat prescribing policy?
- What information is available to patients about the repeat prescribing service?
- How accessible is this information?
- How long does it take patients to get their repeat prescription?
- Who are the patients who are on repeat prescriptions and what do they think about the level of service?
- How often do patients need to contact the practice to get their repeat prescription?
- Does the practice have a system of recording problems that patients experience with their repeats?

For more on repeat prescribing, *see* www.schin.ncl.ac.uk/repeatprescribing.

# Consumer health informatics at the societal level

In some senses, the healthcare professional is outside the scope of this particular form of consumer health informatics as it represents mostly what patients do outside the traditional health service. The Internet

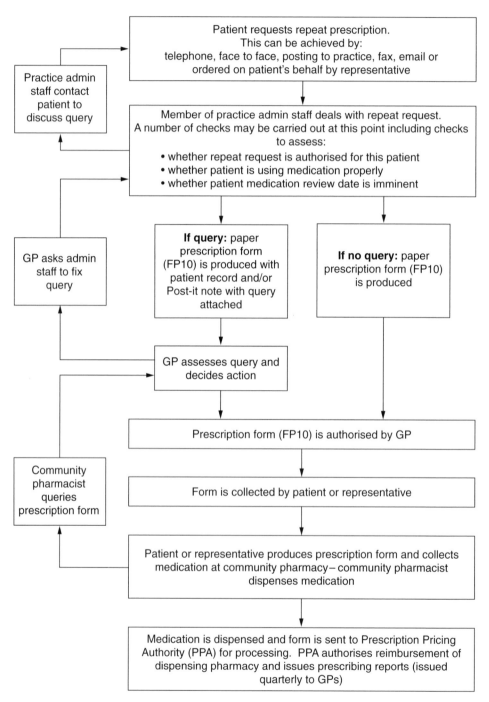

**Figure 7.4**   The key points in the repeat prescription process.

facilitates consumer-to-consumer interaction in a way never seen before and these electronic communities are thriving. The role of patient self-help groups and societies is expanding, as improvements in technology have made running a group economically viable. These trends are leading to a generation of more aware and better-informed patients, who are becoming active in seeking to understand their condition and its effects.

Patient on-line support groups best exemplify subject-centred electronic communities. They deal with a specific subject area – in the case of patients and health professionals usually a chronic disease such as diabetes or cancer. They offer support in a number of forms including:

- information about new products or treatments
- assessment of treatments from a mixture of personal accounts to discussion of scientific evidence
- emotional support network for sufferers of a disease and often their carers.

Although this trend has until now been outside the remit of the UK official health service, the benefits to patients are beginning to be shown to be effective. Two examples from the US are the CHESS project for those with a HIV+ status, which has been proven to support the needs of AIDs health consumers, and the Idaho Healthwise project, which is an ongoing process seeking to educate the health provider and consumer stakeholders with the aim of building a better healthcare system (www.healthwise.org).

## Bringing it together

The aim of this chapter is not to show how consumer health informatics *can* but how it *is* becoming an integral part of consumers' experience of what is their healthcare. Reflecting on the three aspects of consumer health informatics that promote clinical governance, it has been shown that the everyday experiences of the NHS customer can be improved by seeking to improve the core services described. The increase in information should become the catalyst for those giving and receiving care to build a new relationship. High-quality services, care, information, communication and mutual trust are likely to be key. This means getting the basics right, and sharing decisions in consultations, appointment scheduling, repeat prescribing and engaging in dialogue with patients are representative of these requirements.

# Web and other resources

Box 7.1 lists current UK-based projects that provide information or supporting services oriented to health consumers.

# References

1  Eysenbach G (2000) Recent advances: consumer health informatics. *Br Med J* **320**: 1713–16.
2  Jones R, Pearson J, McGregor S *et al.* (1999) Randomised trial of personalised computer based information for cancer patients. *Br Med J* **319**: 1241–7.
3  Kenny T, Wilson R, Purves I *et al.* (1998) A PIL for every ill? Patient information leaflets: a review of past, present and future use. *Family Practice* **15**: 471–9.

**Box 7.1**

| | | |
|---|---|---|
| NHS Direct | This includes the phone service but also a website NHS Direct Online | www.nhsdirect.nhs.uk |
| National Institute for Clinical Excellence (NICE) | NICE produces information for healthcare consumers seeking a short and understandable version of NICE decisions | www.nice.org.uk |
| PRODIGY | Available through the GP computer system, the PRODIGY module actively supports clinical governance in consultations by providing a range of features that can be used to share decisions with the patient and give patients more information through the provision of leaflets | www.prodigy.nhs.uk |
| Centre for Health Information Quality (CHIQ) | The Centre for Health Information Quality seeks to support the provision of high-quality information for patients. Training courses available | www.hfht.org.uk/chiq |
| Patient UK | Produced by Patient Information Publications (PIP), this is a highly regarded site for links to patient groups and organisations that have websites | www.patient.co.uk |
| NHS.UK | Patient-friendly portal for the NHS | www.nhs.uk |
| National Association for Patient Participation | The National Association for Patient Participation is a registered charity providing support and advice to those wishing to start a patient group | www.napp.org.uk |
| Royal Pharmaceutical Society and Concordance Group | Concordance is a new approach to the prescribing and taking of medicines. It is an agreement reached after negotiation between a patient and a healthcare professional. This includes training material for concordance in the consultation | www.concordance.org |
| NHS Modernisation Agency – Patient Access and Primary Care teams | Parts of the agency seeking to support patients and primary care. One current focus is supporting PCOs with NHS Plan appointments targets | www.modernnhs.nhs.uk/ |

# 8

# Showing and reflecting: shop windows and mirrors

*Paul Robinson and Louise Simpson*

---

**Key points covered in this chapter**

- The place of perspective
- SMART goals
- Planning and measuring success
- Shop windows – what have I got and what do I want to show?
- Reflection, learning and appraisal

---

## It depends how you look at it . . .

This chapter is about perspective. Our interpretation of information depends on the perspective from which we view it. When we present information to other people, we have to take into account their perspectives. At the same time, the act of preparing information for presentation to others may alter our own perspectives. The language of this chapter is visual.

One way that computer systems can help with clinical governance and clinical practice is in the presentation of data. Searches, audits and reports are popular uses for clinical computer systems, and data collection and data quality issues – the important bit before searches and reports will be of any use. Lots of resources and activities are available to help you with data quality, and PRIMIS is a good starting point.

'Monitoring of targets' is often referred to in journals and articles about clinical governance, NSFs and other national agendas. Most primary care teams will have the capacity in their existing clinical systems to deliver the data, information and knowledge to both reflect (mirrors) and demonstrate concordance (shop windows).

Just as clinical evidence and medical knowledge can be locked in paper and not find their way to the point of care, so can important data that could help us reflect on our practice and demonstrate our quality. Audit used to be a mammoth task of pulling paper records and making paper notes that would take an age to carry out. If you are assured of the quality of your data, then quality information and knowledge in the form of e-reporting can be a much smoother and easier task.

Now they are so much easier to produce, it is worth thinking about the purpose of reports and audits, and different approaches can offer interesting results. It is also important to think about what you want to measure and what your 'success indicators' are before you start. Measuring everything and therefore capturing everything will not motivate the technophobes! Be SMART.

---

**Box 8.1 Make your data collection and reporting targets:**

- Specific
- Measurable
- Achievable
- Reasonable
- Time-phased

---

So how can informatics support the demonstration of concordance and help us reflect on what we actually do? Remember that service quality and data quality are not the same thing.

---

**Box 8.2 Planning and measuring success – five quick tips:**

- Who is the report for?
- Will I be measuring a series of encounters, an outcome or one-off events?
- Is my definition of success the same as that of my partners?
- Will I repeat the measurement? What percentage improvement do I want to see? What counts as 'improvement'?
- Is there a gap between my perception and the 'reality' of the report? Is it a data quality flaw, did I remember it wrong, or both?

---

# Shop windows

We've used the metaphor of the shop window in the title of this chapter. We will develop the metaphor as we go along, but first consider preparing a report of your work as putting your wares in a shop window. Suppose you have just taken over a handicraft shop; how are you going to show your products to their best advantage? There will be some constraints, such as the location of your shop, the size of the window and so on, but that still leaves you with a lot of choice. In deciding how to go about this you will want to know what the competition is doing, so you'll go down the street to see what they've got on show. You will also want to get some idea about the shoppers; who walks up and down the street? What sorts of things interest them? What is the best way to get their attention (in a positive way)?

There are four factors in play.

1 What I've got.
2 What I want to show.
3 The medium (shop window) in which I'll display.
4 The audience.

The focus of this chapter is the third of these – showing – but the choice of medium and the way you use it will clearly depend on the other three factors.

## *Some examples*

Electronic information systems make it much easier to produce reports and audits, and clinical systems can generate some of these automatically, particularly if they are required universally. The outputs from the clinical systems may be idiosyncratic, and although the information may transfer to standard office software such as Word and Excel, the appearance may be a bit raw. You may therefore wish to modify and supplement the raw materials in different ways, depending on the audience.

## Colleagues within the practice/clinical team

This audience will be familiar with the clinical system and the way you work. This means that an informal presentation with limited explanation will suffice. Email, with the information tabulated in the text or as an attachment, is the obvious medium here. Cumulative records of audits or significant events can be stored on an intranet. There are two cautions though. Email is an informal medium and there is a tendency to take short cuts on the grounds that your readers share your culture and world view; be careful that you are not assuming too much about the readers. Second, the fact that you have posted a document to the intranet does not mean that anyone will look at it (nor that all your colleagues know how to do this). A combination of approaches may help.

## Your patients

Increasingly, the general population is becoming more familiar with computer technology. Some practices, for instance the Well Close Square practice in Berwick (www.wellclosesquare.co.uk), are using web-sites to carry information about how they work. Included on the Well Close Square practice website is a summary of their clinical audits. Clearly there are issues about patient confidentiality, but aggregated anonymous data about an organisation's performance are certainly of public interest. Again you need to be clear about your purpose in sharing this information and sure that you are getting the level of the technical language and formality right.

## Managers or administrators in the larger organisation

Now the tone is more formal and your communication may well be addressing specific targets or policy issues. Here, open technologies such as websites, and to some extent email, are less appropriate and the medium is likely to be an electronic document, perhaps sent by email as an attachment. Of course part of this document may be produced by cutting and pasting from internal documents or from material produced for patients and clients.

## *Cautionary note*

A word of caution: it is tempting to try to save time by presenting information in one format that you hope will be accessible to all your readers. From the point of view of the individual who has links with all the other parties (i.e. you), it is easy to feel sure that everyone will understand your carefully crafted work. You are the least able of anybody to judge this. Much better to adapt your material to each different audience and, if you can, have it read by someone else before posting. The meaning that people put on to the written word is culturally determined and only someone from the relevant culture can interpret the meaning of your writing for that group.

# Shop windows revisited

Let's go back to the window in your new handicraft shop. Time has moved on, you've looked at your stock and decided what you want to display, you've had a look around to see what the competition is doing and you've worked out (more or less) what you want to do. This is fine, but time has moved on and your deadline is tomorrow morning and you are working late. Outside, it's dark; inside, your window space is brightly lit. As you work, moving your stuff around, stopping and thinking, moving it back, you glance up at the big glass pane of the window and you see a reflection of yourself, surrounded by your stuff. Sometimes you will go outside and look in to see what it looks like, but this is a very different view from the reflected image you get from the inside, not least because you are in one view and not the other.

The point about this story is that the process of displaying your wares (i.e. preparing reports for other people to read) is inextricably linked to the process of reflecting on what you have been doing. You reflect on the value of your work, for yourself and for others. The shared reflections are fed back into practice and so improve the quality of practice; this is all part of the clinical governance story.

That is how clinical governance should work. Hopefully it will, but its success depends on practitioners being prepared to share their strengths and development areas openly and honestly. This in turn depends on there being trust between people in different parts of the organisation. This is easy to write but difficult to achieve, and is in conflict with the blame culture that exists in large organisations like the NHS. It is also more difficult for primary care practitioners, who usually work alone with their patient behind a closed door, to share things about their work than it is for practitioners who are used to the more public environment of the hospital ward or outpatient clinic.

|  | Known to me | Not known to me |
|---|---|---|
| Known to others | **Arena** | **Blind spot** |
| Not known to others | **Facade** | **Unknown to self or others** |

**Figure 8.1**  The Johari window.

# Trust

This issue of trust is illustrated by the Johari window (Figures 8.1 and 8.2). The Johari window is a very useful model, and it particularly relates to self-awareness. The working area is called the 'arena'. To the right of this is the person's blind spot: here there are things that he or she does not know about himself or herself but others can see. Below the arena is an area called the 'facade': here the person knows things that he or she is not prepared to share.

The aim of clinical governance is to increase the area of the arena section. The blind spot is reduced by feedback, the facade is increased through disclosure, and these processes of feedback and disclosure are interrelated through trust. If someone gives you honest feedback that rings true, then you will trust them a bit more and so will be prepared to disclose things to them. This then makes it easier for them to give you appropriate feedback and so on. It is clear from this that the relationship between the practitioner and the person who is sharing the information is very important. This is true whether the other person be a colleague, manager, appraiser or confidante.

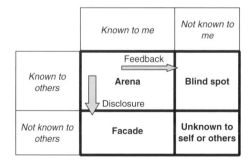

**Figure 8.2**  The Johari window in action.

> **Box 8.3 The Johari window**
>
> - The aim is to increase the size of the arena
> - The blind spot is reduced by **feedback**
> - Facade is reduced by **disclosure**
> - Feedback and disclosure work together and are interdependent
> - Both feedback and disclosure depend on trust

# Learning needs

At the heart of the concept of clinical governance is the idea of bringing learning needs to light, identifying and understanding them, and then meeting them. In the section on lifelong learning in Chapter 3, we mentioned the problems of relating an individual's perceived learning needs to the needs of their organisation and its clients. These problems can be resolved by a period of reflection followed by a discussion with a 'trusted other'. This is the model of appraisal used in the NHS Appraisal Toolkit (www.appraisals.nhs.uk), which we will describe later.

The Johari window lends itself particularly to learning needs. There are needs that you don't know about (blind spot) and ones that you do know about but don't want to acknowledge (facade). We have just described the way that feedback and disclosure work together to increase the shared arena. There is another pair of processes at work here: reflection and presentation. A list of learning needs, which can be formalised into a personal development plan, is a presentation or a display. Everything we said about presentation earlier in this chapter applies here, even though you may be more comfortable with presenting your achievements than your needs.

# Methods of reflection

Different people prefer different methods of reflection. Some people will jot down notes while others may write more formally. Some people will talk things over with colleagues or with their partner, while others may sit and think, or go for a walk. One of the problems with reflection in a busy professional life is that so much is happening that there is no time to think. General practitioners see a new patient every 7 to 10 minutes, and may see 20 or more patients in one session. Where is the time in this sort of schedule to reflect on the action that has taken place? Suppose the fourth patient prompts a question in the practitioner's mind: '*Is there another treatment for this condition? Wasn't there something about this in the* BMJ *last year?*' How likely is it that the task of dealing with the next 15 people will displace these questions from the GP's mind? The questions may then go unanswered and practice remain locked in the existing pattern.

Setting time aside to think, or tell stories, about your work is a key part of professional development. Apart from finding the time to do this, there is the problem of preserving the questions and points of interest that arise in day-to-day work. Some practitioners are in the habit of scribbling notes or memos as they go along, possibly in a book or notepad, possibly on bits of paper that may get lost or buried. How much easier to keep a tabulated record on the desktop computer!

An on-line group of GPs have been working through these issues of learning needs and learning portfolios, and they are developing electronic methods of producing personal development plans. You can find out more about their work from their website (www.wisdomnet.co.uk).

## The NHS Appraisal Toolkit

The NHS Appraisal Toolkit (www.appraisals.nhs.uk) is an on-line resource to support the appraisal of GPs in the first instance, but the concepts and format will apply to other professional groups in the NHS. Appraisal can become a once-a-year process that is helpful at the time, but forgotten for the next 11 months until the next round is due. The NHS Appraisal Toolkit is built around a questionnaire that addresses different aspects of the practitioner's work. There are different tools that support reflection, 'my notes' areas that serve as notepads, and the questionnaire itself can be edited and text can be pasted in from other sources. This design of the NHS Appraisal Toolkit, and the fact that it is available through NHSNet or other Internet connection on the practitioner's desktop, means that it can be accessed at any time through the year. So it will support immediate reflection on events as well as more measured and (possibly) leisurely reflection on work.

## Some final thoughts

This chapter has been built round the metaphor of displaying your wares in a shop window and based on the idea that display and reflection are twin processes that are intertwined – two sides of the same coin. Putting the spotlight on part of your life reveals it to you as well as to others. In particular, the process of preparing your display informs you. The sheet of glass is the interesting thing here: look at it and you may just see glass (or at least the flaws in it and the dust on it); the view through it; or your own reflection. Which you see is a matter of choice, focus and lighting.

Preparing a formal written report, such as an appraisal statement or a personal development plan, casts light on both you and the reader. It will change both you and the organisation you work in. It's been the same for us writing this chapter: it has made us think and look at ourselves, and so has changed us and the way we think.

# 9

# The clinical computer system and e-clinical governance

*Jane Cartridge*

---

**Key points covered in this chapter**

- Meeting the information needs of e-clinical governance
- How data become information
- Data management and the data set
- Principles of data searching

---

This chapter is essentially about data management, but before you move quickly onwards, let us consider how data management supports the wide range of activities encompassed by clinical governance.

The NHS Clinical Governance Support Team[1] have stated that healthcare in the 21st century should be:

- patient-centred
- accountable
- systematic
- sustained.

And that clinical governance is committed to the pursuit of best practice in the following areas:

- clinical technique
- risk management
- patient experience
- communication excellence
- effective resourcing
- strategic implementation
- quality learning.

Accountability is self-evidently a good reason for keeping records. However, all the above aspects of healthcare and best practice are accessible to measurement and assessment to a greater or lesser degree. This can provide evidence of progress towards, or achievement of, gold standards of practice across the range of general medical services, service development, and, increasingly, monitoring and meeting NSF milestones.

Scally,[2] in a report for Bristol NHSE, drew up a 15-point framework for the implementation of clinical governance, a primary requirement of which was a baseline assessment of clinical quality. Such an assessment is so obviously necessary it hardly needs stating, but it demonstrates the broad impact that clinical governance has on primary care and many of its demands are data hungry. The very statement 'baseline assessment of clinical quality' carries a burden of data requirements which increases with every passing thought. Should this baseline assessment be applied to every possible patient interaction? Is it possible to differentiate between clinical encounters and non-clinical? Does the measurement of clinical care extend to the availability of care through ready access to doctors and nurses in the primary care setting? Within the compass of clinical governance, PCOs will be expected to monitor the performance of their practices and to be able to make comparisons between them. To do this they must be able to draw on reliable data from the practices and to assemble it in a meaningful form.

Some PCOs are seeking to meet these data requirements by commissioning external data collection and bespoke software. Rather than generating fresh data collection initiatives consider which needs can be met by harvesting existing data – data that could be readily available within the primary care clinical systems, collected on a day-to-day basis as part of the normal work of the primary care team. The clinical systems generally provide excellent functions to support data management and report generation. These functions can be utilised either as customised regular searches or ad hoc searches, or by using the suite of reports and the audit facilities provided by the system supplier. As is the case with most software applications, it is a rare user indeed who uses more than a fraction of the power of the clinical computer system, and this would be a fruitful area to explore.

However, and there is always a proviso, for them to be useful at even the most basic level the data must be available, complete, reliable and up-to-date. This chapter aims to elucidate appropriate data collection and offer some suggestions about information management.

## Data and information

Initially let us note that although data can exist in many forms, throughout this chapter it will be assumed that all data are eventually stored on a computer and that data management will rely totally on computerised manipulation.

Data have no value in and of themselves. They must be collected for a clearly defined purpose and that purpose must be transparent to the people who are collecting them as this will enable them to collect and record the data intelligently. Ideally, the collectors themselves will benefit from the data collection, because if this benefit is poor and primary benefit is seen to apply very much higher up the organisation, they may be poorly motivated to comply with requests for data. As the main data providers, the primary care teams will need support and motivation to create and maintain adequate computerised records. Some GPs are learning to use their clinical systems effectively for this purpose, often using PRODIGY (*see* Chapters 2 and 5) to facilitate data collection in a structured and meaningful way within the consultation, and MIQUEST (see later in this chapter) to facilitate data retrieval and analysis. Both of these are provided as part of GP clinical systems under RFA99.

In 1995, Smith[3] differentiated data from information:

'Data is information stripped of its potential value. Data is random fact, whilst information is the ability to earn (or learn) from such random facts.'

Smith goes on to state that:

'Information in short must be appropriate but that is a complication in itself, because even appropriacy (sic) is relative. It varies with the managerial level concerned.'

Drawing on earlier studies from the 1960s he stratifies information in the following way: operational information, tactical information and strategic information.

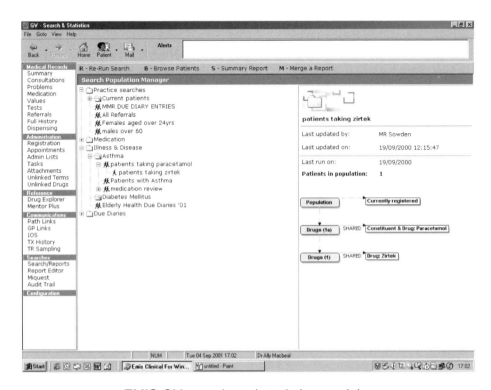

EMIS GV search and statistics module.

## Operational information

This is information needed by those at the bottom of the corporate hierarchy (in our case the primary care team). It is detailed information relating to day-to-day activities – level 1 data.

## Tactical information

This is information needed by those part way up the corporate hierarchy (in our case the PCO or HA). It is frequently a summary of the level 1 information and is often termed 'derived data'.

## Strategic information

This is information needed by those at the top of the corporate hierarchy (in our case, for instance, the Department of Health). It is highly abstracted and summarised and typically relates to the organisation as a whole rather than to its individual divisions.

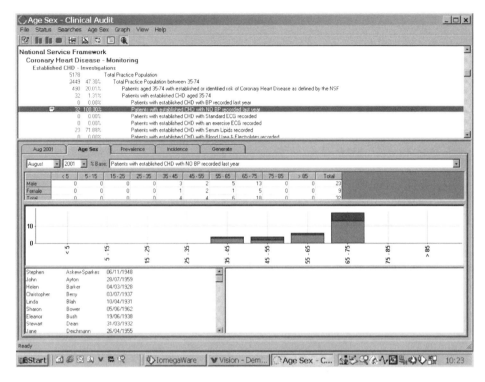

In Practice Systems clinical audit module.

## *Derived data*

This is usually aggregated from lower-level data. The aggregation can be over one or more aspects, but often over time periods and/or a number of age bands. Another popular aggregation is over a particular single diagnosis or group of diagnoses. It is best if the base or lower-level data are collected by those to whom they are relevant, so for individual patients, GPs will be collecting diagnostic data, nurses chronic disease management data and practice managers appointment waiting times, for instance. It is the computer's task to aggregate the data to provide the necessary reports for such things as the number of males over 65 with a diagnosis of depressive illness taking antidepressants.

There is a strong case to be made for entry of basic (level 1) data on to the system at the point of service by the person responsible for the data collection. However, if data are accurately Read coded (see later in this chapter), for instance by the GP on a hospital letter, they could well be entered into the system by a member of the administrative staff. This begs the question of how the GP decides on an accurate Read Code. There may be a recommended list of codes provided by the PCO or created within the

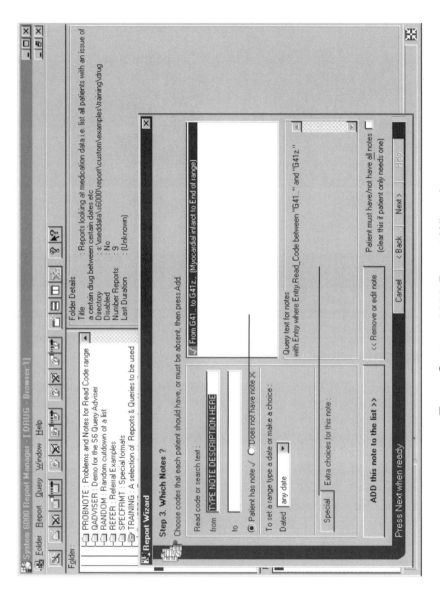

Torex System 6000 Report Wizard.

practice; this is likely to be a paper list, which is easy to refer to but becomes rapidly dog-eared and elusive. If no such list exists and the GP or nurse has to rely on memory, then it is likely that a very limited number of codes will be used and there is a real danger of miscoding or not coding pieces of data at all. The obvious and easy answer is that the person coding the data also enters them on to the system and uses the inbuilt Read Code browser in the clinical system. The important points are the accuracy of the coding and its entry on to the system; one is of little use without the other.

## *Some problems with data collection*

A real difficulty with data collection at the point of service is the observed phenomenon that, because increasing expertise denigrates data collection over pattern recognition, experts gather less, rather than more, data than their juniors.[4] In primary care this is reflected in some GPs 'knowing my patients' response' in many situations of potential change.

This section was entitled 'Data and information'. At what point do the data become information? At its simplest, data become information when they become useable. Implicit in this usability is the application of intelligence to the data to interpret them. A BP reading recorded on the computer is a data item within its storage system. When that reading appears on screen as part of the patient record it becomes information. Being able to understand or make use of information converts it to knowledge. Some data will never be information on their own, only when aggregated with other data and perhaps only following statistical analysis. Relevant, reliable data are the building blocks of all information.

## Knowledge and wisdom

We have compared data with information. Before we move on to the practicalities of data collection and information management, let us look at the following extrapolation from data to wisdom.[5]

Data on their own have no meaning; only when interpreted by some kind of data processing system do they take on meaning and become information.

People or computers can find patterns in data to perceive information and information can be used to enhance knowledge. Since knowledge is a prerequisite to wisdom, we always want more data and information.

- '1234567.89' is data.
- 'Your bank balance has jumped 8087% to £1234567.89' is information.
- 'Nobody owes me that much money' is knowledge.
- 'I'd better talk to the bank before I spend it, because of what has happened to other people' is wisdom.

# Data collection in the primary care team

*It is a truth universally acknowledged that a GP in possession of a computer must be in want of training.*

## Read Codes

Coordinated by the NHS Information Authority, Read Codes are supplied as an integral part of GP clinical systems. Read Codes were adopted in 1988 as the standard for general practice computing. They are compiled and updated regularly (quarterly for general codes and monthly for drugs). The Read Codes comprise a list of terms that healthcare professionals in primary care can use to describe the care and treatment of their patients. Read Codes allow practices to:

- record data more consistently
- retrieve data with greater ease
- analyse and audit data more thoroughly
- communicate data to other agencies.

The Read Codes cover a wide range of topics in categories such as signs and symptoms, treatments and therapies, investigations, occupations, diagnoses, and drugs and appliances. The descriptive part of the code (preferred term, synonym or rubric) is in naturalistic clinical language. The code part is an alpha-numeric four- or five-digit code (depending on the version). In the most recent version (version 3), all characters in the range a–z, A–Z and 0–9 are available, giving a theoretical number of codes of 916,132,832. Such a huge number of codes will never be practically useful. Indeed the Scottish Clinical Information Management in Primary Care offers a list of 300 'core codes' and a list of 800 'complete codes'[6] that it considers adequate to meet the current requirements of clinical governance.

Read Codes are structured in a hierarchy or tree-like structure in which

| Table 9.1 Read Code hierarchy | | |
|---|---|---|
| *Preferred term* | *Code* | |
| Circulatory disease | G | The highest level code |
| Ischaemic heart disease | G3 | Second level |
| Acute myocardial infarction | G30 | Third level |
| Anterior myocardial infarction NOS | G301 | Fourth level |
| Acute anteroseptal infarction | G3011 | Fifth level |

overarching or high-level codes branch out into more detailed codes, as in Table 9.1.

The code G30 is parent to the code G3011. This is pertinent to the search strategies you can undertake (see data retrieval section). There is a wealth of information on the Web describing and critiquing Read Codes.[7] Any clinical computing system has a full Read Code browser.

### A note about SNOMED

You may have heard about SNOMED. These clinical terms will cover not only primary care but all healthcare, including medicine, nursing and the professions allied to medicine. This new system is necessary to implement the electronic patient record (EPR) and electronic health record (EHR) and will provide a platform for international communication and analysis. Guidance will be issued on the timetable for implementation of SNOMED within the NHS.[8]

## The scope and range of data collection

*A single unit of data is a data item. A data item has a value of some sort (e.g. a number of years in an age, hair colour, a Read Code). A data item is an individual observation, it cannot be broken down. A computer uses a database to store data. This assembly of data items is known as a dataset.*

The simplest way to assess the scope of a clinical computer database is to look at one. It can record with a Read Code every visit to the consulting room, every phone call, every blood test and cervical smear, every diagnosis and every tear shed, every prescription issued, every pregnancy, lab tests, items of service and appointments for every one of the patients on the list.

It doesn't matter how much data the GP records so long as he or she records the items you need. As we saw earlier, some organisations are controlling the recording of data by issuing a list of Read Codes. So a list may define a set of codes at levels 2 and 3 to capture data to match the requirements of the NSF disease registers. The decision must then be taken whether Read Coding is to be carried out retrospectively or as patients present for consultation. Retrospective coding is resource intensive but relatively speedy. Practices may feel able to do this in-house or PCOs may favour providing external resources to ensure completion of the task throughout its constituent practices.

Even those GPs who record abundant data may be recording the data in such a way that they are inaccessible to the computer. For instance, BP measurements can be and should be recorded as a Read Code, which enables it to be used by the system, for example to show in graphical format the patient's BP measurements over time. Coded data items can be retrieved by the system to enable computerised decision support within the consultation either by the host system or by PRODIGY. However, because they do not thoroughly (or indeed at all) understand the way in which data are stored, many GPs record information as free text which cannot be searched for or used by the system. Free text is of use only to the person looking at the patient record on the screen. It is self-evident that if data aren't there you won't be able to find them, but for someone who is untrained in the ways of computerised data storage it is difficult to understand that information on the screen is not necessarily visible to the computer itself.

The majority of GPs issue both acute and repeat prescriptions by computer and therefore drug and prescription data will be largely complete and up to date. There will be a small proportion of scripts not accounted for – those that were hand written on domiciliary visits. Controlled drug scripts may not be on the computer, although in many cases they are issued by computer and later destroyed when a hand-written version is obtained; in this case the computer retains the record.

Most practices use the appointment system included in the clinical system. These data are probably already used by the practice manager to audit surgery size and failure to attend. In addition, this information can be included in the GP's personal development plan to demonstrate workload.

Every patient on the GP's list has full personal information stored in the computer. Data items immediately obvious for use are age, sex and postcode.

If the practice is paperless or paper-frugal, every patient will have at least diagnoses recorded on the system. Practices more advanced in computerisation will be recording BP, lab tests, weight, height, health promotion, cervical cytology, contraception and childhood vaccinations.

They will be using the patient record to trigger call and recall for health screening and chronic disease management. Some practices Read Code hospital letters and enter the codes on to the patient record.

These are just examples of the sort of data that is already stored in the computerised patient record. Read Codes are very comprehensive and almost anything you can think of can be Read Coded – a sample from the tip of a catheter for lab culture is code X7AFf. We could not think of anything more obscure, but are sure there's a code for it if we did!

# Data retrieval

This section is not intended to give you step-by-step instructions to using any specific clinical computer system. Rather it is to give you an overview of the sorts of things you can reasonably expect to carry out using the clinical computer alone without the necessity for third-party software.

Deciding what your data requirements are is the most basic step in specifying the data set you need. So knowing what you want to retrieve controls what you want to record. And record reliably. This reliability really only needs to be a level 3 (*see* Table 9.1), unless you are pursuing a specialised piece of research. If all you want to know is the number of women in your area with angina, then it is irrelevant how many Prinzmetal anginas have been recorded by the GPs. Because of the structure of the Read Codes you would simply search for records at the level of G33 and all anginas will be returned. But if you need to know about those Prinzmetals then you must be sure that everyone knows (a) that they need to record it, and (b) that they can find it in the Read Code browser even if they have forgotten how to spell it. Simply typing in angina will bring up the full list of various anginas from which to choose.

At its simplest level data in the clinical systems can be interrogated using the inbuilt query or search functions of the system. All systems will provide a set of predetermined searches that will return data either in their raw form or as a predesigned report. This is not to imply that the queries are simplistic. They are often designed to allow practices to carry out clinical audit activities. If the search required is not included in the system suite, it is a straightforward task to build ad hoc or customised regular queries. These queries or searches can become quite complex if the principles of searching are adhered to. It is likely that you will want to define a population and elicit the frequency of a variable or compare frequencies over time. Prevalence of a variable (e.g. diagnosis) within a defined population is also a common requirement. Queries such as one comparing the number of patients with coronary heart disease

(CHD) and those receiving anti-platelet therapy are frequently performed. It is possible to break down the data to demonstrate what
therapy is being prescribed, e.g. to show who is receiving clopidogrel
without aspirin.

Essentially you must know what you want to find and what you want
not to find. There may be more than one way of expressing the criteria in
any individual system.

---

To find the number of men over the age of 65 prescribed tricyclic
antidepressants in the last six months and with a diagnosis of
depressive illness:

- Exclude age $< 65$ (this could be shown as Include age $\geq 65$)
- Exclude female (this could be shown as Include male)
- Include BNF section 4.3.1
- Between dates [today's date] and [six months ago]
- Include Problem code E204
- Apply to today's practice population (this will exclude deceased
  patients)

---

Using the same basic design you could return those men on tricyclics who
do **not** have a diagnosis of depressive illness nor of arthritis (in which
tricyclics are sometimes being prescribed for pain relief) and ascertain
whether their prescription is appropriate.

---

- Exclude problem code E204
- Exclude problem code N050

---

It may simply turn up coding omissions, of course!

The results of a query will be displayed on screen in a variety of formats,
such as frequency tables collated by age and sex; a linear graph; a bar
chart; a list of patients with a selection of demographic data. The systems
will have an inbuilt reports function which may allow you to design your
own output. The quality of the result will depend on which printer is
used; the prescription printer will be quick and cheap but not suitable for
transmission to a third party nor for inclusion in a report. Data can usually
be exported at the click of a mouse to MSExcel where they can have a
range of statistical and mathematical functions applied to them. MSExcel
is capable of producing such things as pivot tables and a range of
graphical outputs that are highly manipulable.

Some examples of using the search or query facilities in clinical computing systems have been shown in this chapter. If you have specific data collection or extraction needs that are not easily met by existing facilities it is worthwhile contacting the clinical system suppliers with your request. It may be that they can elucidate which part of the system will meet your needs or perhaps provide some specialised help in constructing a data entry guideline or template.

If the practices across a PCO use the same system, then data collection and comparison is a relatively simple matter, but you may prefer the support of PRIMIS to assist you in progressing your analytical work. Where data from different systems are to be analysed then a third party is required. MIQUEST is now provided as part of RFA99-approved clinical systems. Some GPs are using this themselves to extract data from their system but the analytical work is undertaken by PRIMIS (Primary Care Information Services). Information about both MIQUEST and PRIMIS is available from the NHS Information Authority or on the Web at www.clinical-info.co.uk/miquest.htm for MIQUEST and www.primis. nottingham.ac.uk for PRIMIS. MIQUEST is a Health Query Language which is able to work with commonly used GP clinical systems and has been successfully utilised by several health authorities and practices in England and Wales for projects ranging from health needs assessment to practice-based research. It allows the collection of aggregated, anonymous data from GP clinical computer systems. It can be used for regular queries, ad hoc enquiries, continuous data collection, populating research data-bases and following cohorts of patients.

PRIMIS is a support service that is free of charge to PCOs (funded by the NHS Information Authority). It specialises in promoting effective use of GP clinical computer systems. It provides training and support in information management skills, data recording, extraction and analysis.

*Illustrations provided by, and used with permission from, Torex Health,[9] EMIS[10] and In Practice Systems.[11]*

# References

1   Clinical Governance Support Team (www.cgsupport.org).
2   Scally G (2000) *Clinical Governance Annual Report 1999/2000.* NHS Executive, Bristol.
3   Smith D (1995) *System Engineering for Healthcare Professionals.* Half module 216 workbook. Cardiff Institute of Higher Education, Cardiff.
4   Schmidt and Norman (1990) Cited in R Beaumont (1997) *Introduction to Health Informatics for Specialist Registrars.* SCHIN, Newcastle University.

5  FOLDOC – Free Online Dictionary of Computing (http://wombat.doc.ic. ac.uk/).
6  Clinical Effectiveness Programme in Practice-based Primary Care (www.ceppc.org/scimp/readcodeindex.shtml).
7  CAMS (www.cams.co.uk/readcode.htm); Structural and lexical features of successive versions of the Read Codes (www.phcsg.org.uk/conferences/ camb96/readcode.htm); Oxford Medical Informatics (www.oxmedinfo.jr2.ox. ac.uk/wwwdocs/read/readinfov2.html).
8  www.coding.nhsia.nhs.uk/clin_term/snomedct.asp
9  www.torexhealth.co.uk
10  www.emis-online.co.uk
11  www.inps.co.uk

# 10

# Education and training for e-clinical governance

*Louise Simpson*

---

**Key points covered in this chapter**

- Making it happen, bringing it all to life

- What is training for?

- Principles of adult learning

- Barriers to change

- Some examples of education and training resources

---

## Making it happen

We are now getting to the end of this stage in the journey towards e-clinical governance. We have seen that the main challenge is to know what is possible. Now we can look at how to make it happen. We have shown throughout this book that there are many aspects of clinical governance that can be supported and delivered by utilising the magic of informatics and exploiting the investment you make in your clinical computer system. Finally, therefore, a word about training.

# What is training for?

Training is one technique in the management and introduction of change. We looked at tacit and explicit knowledge acquisition in Chapter 2, and training is another part of the change management toolkit. A range of training strategies can be brought to bear – group work, one-to-one training, computer-based sessions and so on. You will know what suits you, and we hope this book has shown you some areas where it might be worth investing some time to investigate further. Intensive one-day training courses are not the only option, but contacting your clinical system supplier to see what they have to offer might be a good step. Persuading everyone in a practice to set aside a whole afternoon for training is often difficult, and you may choose to adopt a cascade method, but make sure it is executed appropriately. The person who understands the wiring inside the grey box is not necessarily the best person to be your dedicated cascade trainer.

# Principles of adult learning

Adult learning principles propose ideas of involving the student in the planning and evaluation of their training, and utilising students' experiences as a basis for learning. This is not the same as 'doing what I feel like doing'; the importance of reflection to correctly identify learning needs is key here.

# Barriers to change

There is a wealth of literature on barriers to behaviour change, and expositions on why it can happen that professional training, CME and consulting colleagues can improve knowledge and skill, but not patient care. One of the simplest – and most effective – ways to identify the barriers is to talk to the prospective learner and really get behind what he or she is saying. Does the rejection of the computer system because 'it takes too long in a seven-minute consultation' actually reflect poor familiarity with what is appearing on the screen, so it *seems* to take much longer? Does it show the learners' anxiety about losing rapport with the patient? The better training programmes take these anxieties into account and not only show how they can be overcome, but will also demonstrate how rapport, for example, might be improved.

# Some examples of training resources

This is not an exhaustive list of the resources available for exploring the possible training options. Many practices and PCOs will have training and education leads who may offer a rewarding insight into the available options as a first port of call.

## Clinical system supplier training

Research carried out at SCHIN suggested that practices that had on-site training from their clinical system supplier are the practices most likely to embrace and take up using different modules of their computer system. Good clinical system supplier trainers are worth their weight in gold, and will know the software inside out. Their insight into primary care is often invaluable, as they can help identify and map your training needs while sharing best practice. A good trainer will have developed a relationship with your practice and locality over time and will be as proficient in facilitation skills as he or she is at making the software jump through hoops (if this is not your experience of clinical system supplier training, contact your supplier and make sure they know so they can do something about it). The trainer is often a vital link between you and the company, so make the most of them. Training from suppliers might be modular and off-the-shelf or it might be tailor-made, but both should come with full supporting training materials and user guides. Discounts are usually available for block bookings across a locality, so it's worth exploring this type of training at PCO as well as practice level.

## National and local clinical system user groups

There is nothing quite as helpful as finding out what colleagues do and how they tackle specific issues, whether it be applying informatics to clinical governance or how to implement the appointments module. Most major clinical systems have active national user groups, usually offering a useful magazine, annual conference, website and representation to the company as a minimum. Contact yours to see what else is available to help you develop your clinical system use. Many national groups have a network of local groups that meet regularly, often at a practice, and share ideas, showing 'how we do it at our place'. Priceless.

## Prodigy *National Dissemination Office (education and training programme)*

The days of launching a software module, such as the Prodigy computer-based decision support programme, *without* a supporting education, communications and training programme are over, we hope. Because Prodigy is built into existing clinical computer systems, it has the look and feel of your usual software. The accompanying Prodigy education and training programme – funded by the Department of Health, currently free of charge – offers 30-minute, one-to-one training to GPs within signed-up PCG/Ts. For the technophobe, 30 minutes – at their own desk in their own consulting room – is a much more comfortable (and likely!) option than giving up a half-day to that scary grey box. To the regular computer user, 30 minutes is all it takes to learn the Prodigy ropes. Your usual system supplier trainer, who has been accredited by the Prodigy team from the University of Newcastle, delivers the training. The trainer will not only cover the key-presses, but also look at some of the concepts and barriers to individual use of Prodigy and using the computer in the consulting room. More information is available from the Prodigy National Dissemination Office or *see* www.prodigy.nhs.uk.

## PRIMIS

Data quality is one of the foundation stones to information proficiency, and this well-established and useful programme would be a good starting point. *See* www.primis.org.uk.

## HIP for CHD

The HIP project – health informatics programme for the coronary heart disease National Service Framework – describes itself as a 'practical example of clinical governance'. HIP for CHD aims to offer a practical and team-based approach, engendering the skills, software tools, knowledge base and organisational structure for a practice or PCO to successfully deliver the CHD NSF. *See* www.hipforchd.org.uk.

## NHS Clinical Governance Support Team

The RAID model is key to this education and training programme, which addresses the implementation of clinical governance, culture and the management of change within an organisation. *See* www.nhscgst.org.uk.

## NHS Information Authority 'Ways of Working' Programme

The aim of the NHSIA 'WoW' programme is to support local NHS organisations to plan and coordinate their education, training and development through two national programmes – 'Developing the right skills' and 'Finding the right help'. Each region has an information education, training and development adviser whose job it is to spread good practice. *See* www.nhsia.nhs.uk/wowwi.

# Index